Judith Wills is one of the country's most popular diet and fitness writers. She has a weekly slimming column in the *Daily Express* and is a regular broadcaster on TV and radio.

Also available in Sphere Books by Judith Wills:

HIGH SPEED SLIMMING

A
Flat Stomach
in
FIFTEEN DAYS

by

Judith Wills

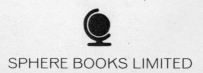

SPHERE BOOKS LIMITED

A SPHERE Book

First published in Great Britain by Sphere Books 1990
Reprinted 1990 (four times)
2nd edition 1991
Reprinted 1991 (twice)

Copyright © Judith Wills 1990, 1991
Exercise photographs © Harry Ormesher 1990
Back cover photograph © Tony Allen 1990

Black and white leotard courtesy of branches of
The Dance Bizarre, London NW3

Typeset by Leaper & Gard Ltd, Bristol, England
Printed and bound in Great Britain by
Cox & Wyman Ltd, Reading

ISBN 0 7474 0959 5

Sphere Books Ltd
A Division of
Macdonald & Co (Publishers) Ltd
165 Great Dover Street
London SE1 4YA
A member of Maxwell Macmillan Publishing Corporation

Contents

Introduction

Ever since *A Flat Stomach in 15 Days* was first published a year ago, I've been getting letters.

'I was so happy to find your book at last — the only system that has really improved my stomach and waist almost overnight.'

'I found the diet advice as effective as the exercises.'

'I gave the programme total effort as you asked — and it *did* work. Thanks so much.'

'All the family enjoy the recipes — and I'm thrilled with my new figure. An hour or so a week keeps it in trim.'

'I thought my stomach was a hopeless case — nothing worked until now. Your book could have saved me years of feeling self-conscious about my body. So why didn't you write it sooner?!'

Why indeed? I devised the Flat Stomach Programme in 1989 for selfish reasons — I was in dire need of a stomach and waist reshape myself. You see, I am not and never have been a Jane Fonda or a Raquel Welch — I'm not a professional exerciser. Although I have spent the last fifteen years or so helping weight-conscious Britons sort out what's rot and what's not in the world of diet and fitness, and although I have rarely been more than a few pounds overweight, when it came to EXERCISE, my policy had always been, 'Don't do as I do — do as I say.'

I know what it's like to search in vain for a dress that fits size 12 bust and hips but will also cater for a size 16 middle. I, too, have pondered on the unfairness of life when the legs on all the jeans in the shop fit perfectly — but none of the zips will do up. And I have been mortified at being congratulated on my pregnancy when I had the baby months ago.

I can also fully sympathise with every one of the millions of men who has to struggle every morning with the momentous decision — shall he belt his trousers *over the top* of his pot belly, or, with difficulty, *across the middle* of it, or once again settle for boring *underneath*?

Believe it — there is nothing you can tell me about the nightmare of a fat middle that I don't already know. Even as a skinny teenager, I had a stomach that defied all my efforts to keep it in line with the rest of my profile. Then in my twenties, thanks, I suppose, to idleness and hours slumped over a typewriter, my stomach expanded further and my waist kindly disappeared, too. In my thirties, two pregnancies did the final damage.

Though I can't have been more than half a

stone overweight, eighteen months ago my waist measured a quite amazing 32″ and my stomach was 35″. And yes I do have the ghastly photos to remind me.

My husband began to make jokes about borrowing my spare tyre for his car. I looked *awful* in swimsuits, leotards and all clingy clothes. Lycra didn't so much hold me in as squash me out. I looked even worse in bikinis and briefs, appalling in all straight skirts, and couldn't even look at anything with a belt.

The truth is that a less-than-perfect middle can ruin an otherwise-perfect figure, and that conversely if you err on the large side, reducing your stomach and waist can instantly change you from looking *big* to looking *curvy* (if you happen to be female). And if you happen to be male, incidentally, I believe that inside every pot-bellied, saddlebag-waisted man is a size 30″ Levi guy just waiting to get out.

Let's face it — we all agree that a sleek, firm, flat stomach and a tight waistline to go with it is what we really want. Consumer surveys have shown me that four out of five people hate their middles. And *A Flat Stomach in 15 Days* is the simple answer for everyone.

I had tried several exercise regimes over the years, but none had made more than a marginal difference to my stomach and waist. I began to feel that I was stuck with this shape. Then I realised the solution — instead of trying other people's methods, I would do what I had done once before. As a diet columnist and editor of a slimming magazine, when I hadn't been able to find a user-friendly diet to help me shed a stone after my last pregnancy, I had devised my own, and it had worked first for me and then for thousands of other people.

I would do the same for my shape. I would devise the ultimate flat stomach programme — for me and for you.

It had to be simple (who can, and who wants to, memorise complicated routines?). It had to start off easy (otherwise how would I — unsupple, untoned — do it?). But it would have to get progressively harder (otherwise it wouldn't work). Lastly, it had to show quick results (or I would get discouraged). I also knew from experience that what I ate always seemed to have a drastic effect on how my stomach looked, so I knew that the right diet would play a big part.

And eventually with research, trial and error, and a large dose of common sense, the Flat Stomach Programme was finished. Diet and exercise — plus some easy lifestyle and posture modifications: the right combination that gave me that flat stomach at last — over 3″ off my belly and a waist a whole 5″ smaller than it used to be. And thanks to the Positive-Neutral-Negative way of eating, I find it easier than ever before to maintain my weight at around 9 stone 2 lbs.

Now let the programme work for you. Anyone can have a stomach flatter than they ever thought possible and a firmer, neater waist. You'll see a tremendous difference even after a few days, and a remarkable improvement in fifteen days. All I ask is that you read the programme carefully, and follow it faithfully and with dedication. However flabby or saggy or fat your stomach has been — you *can* beat it.

The exercise programme is safe — I made sure of that. You can do it whether you have been a keen exerciser until recently, or have done little, like me, for years. That's because each of the six stomach exercises is graded. You start off on Grade 1, the easiest grade, then when you've mastered that you move to Grade 2, then to 3. That way you do the right amount of work for you. The programme is also pleasant, easy to master and needs no special equipment. All it takes is around 30-40 minutes a day. And, when you're the shape you want to be, it will take you little more than an hour a week to keep that way.

The Positive-Neutral-Negative diet — while totally unique in concept — is uncomplicated and healthy. It caters both for people who need to lose weight (men can lose up to 10 lbs and women up to 7 lbs in the fifteen days) and for people who don't.

Remember all I ask is that you give me your

best effort *every* day while you are on the programme. Promise? I have done the rest.

Then you can look forward to wearing the swimsuits and clothes you could never wear before — maybe in a smaller size than you ever dreamed possible. You'll have extra confidence. And, as a marvellous bonus, the programme has all kinds of health benefits. For instance, it can help, even cure, low back pain, shoulder tension, digestive and bowel troubles and period problems.

I did it. Thousands of others have done it. You can too — it's easy when you know how. So let's turn the page and get started!

CHAPTER ONE

Causes and Cures

Why *is* it that we have such a problem keeping our stomachs in trim?

It is by no means confined to people who could do with losing weight. In fact on a slim person a tubby tum can look even more pronounced. Neither is the problem restricted to women who've had several children, or men who drink too much beer.

You can look at a dozen fit, slim young people with not an ounce of flab on their arms or bottoms or legs — but they're fat round the middle. I've seen top models on the catwalk — even in the swimwear catalogues — with it. Even top athletes and sports-men with it (and I'm not just talking about darts players here!).

'So what?' some people might say. 'Does it really matter if our bellies stick out a bit?' I think it does. Because a fat stomach is not just unsightly and unfashionable — it could well be a symptom of one or more physical problems that need your attention. Cure the stomach, cure the problems, and you'll be a healthier person as well as a happier one.

So let's look at what could be the reasons for

your big stomach. For without the cause — or, in this case, causes — we can't find the cure.

1. IS IT FAT?

Your bulging stomach is only likely to be totally due to a layer of surplus fat if you are overweight. In other words, if you are carrying too much fat *all over*.

It is true that women have a natural tendency to accumulate fat around the hips and thighs (that's okay for the nineties!) and on the stomach to a lesser extent. But this layer of fat should simply be an unobtrusive continuation of the rounded line on the hips. The fat should be flat, in other words, not a sudden bulge on the lower abdomen. You should be able to place a rule or stick on the front pelvic bone at either side below your waist and, even allowing for a fat layer, your stomach should offer the rule no resistance.

So, if you're not overweight yet you don't pass this test, don't blame it all on fat. If you've ever *been* overweight, or if you are one of those women who tends to store more fat across her middle than most of us, I must say very loudly and clearly that the answer is *not* to try dieting even more. All that will happen is that you will get thinner all over — but in all probability your body profile will still not be flat. You *cannot* (whatever you may have read

HEIGHT/WEIGHT CHART FOR WOMEN

Height	Average weight	Acceptable weight range
4ft 11ins	104lbs	94-122lbs
1.5 metres	47.25kgs	42.75-55.5kgs
5ft 0ins	107lbs	96-125lbs
1.52 metres	48.75kgs	44-57kgs
5ft 1in	110lbs	99-128lbs
1.55 metres	50kgs	45-58kgs
5ft 2ins	113lbs	102-131lbs
1.57 metres	51.5kgs	46.5-59.5kgs
5ft 3ins	116lbs	105-134lbs
1.60 metres	52.75kgs	47.75-61kgs
5ft 4ins	120lbs	108-138lbs
1.62 metres	54.5kgs	49-62.75kgs
5ft 5ins	123lbs	111-142lbs
1.65 metres	56kgs	50.5-64.5kgs
5ft 6ins	128lbs	114-146lbs
1.67 metres	58kgs	52-66kgs
5ft 7ins	132lbs	118-150lbs
1.70 metres	60kgs	54-68kgs
5ft 8ins	136lbs	122-154lbs
1.73 metres	61kgs	55.5-70kgs
5ft 9ins	140lbs	126-158lbs
1.75 metres	63.5kgs	57-72kgs
5ft 10ins	144lbs	130-163lbs
1.78 metres	65.5kgs	59-74kgs
5ft 11ins	148lbs	134-168lbs
1.80 metres	67kgs	61-76kgs

to the contrary) spot-reduce *fat* on a particular area of your body by going on a low-calorie diet. Your body doesn't know where you're hoping to lose the weight from — it's not that clever. So, if you're not overweight, low-calorie diets are OUT.

Are you overweight? Check on the chart on page 9. There is no such thing as an ideal weight, accurate to the last pound — but if your weight tends towards the upper end of the 'average' shown, you could be overweight. If you're out of the 'acceptable' range altogether, you should slim. You can still follow my programme — as you lose weight, it will ensure your flat stomach at the end of the diet.

If you just go on a low-calorie diet without my programme, you may find that you reach target — but your stomach doesn't!

2. IS IT WEAK STOMACH MUSCLES?

I would say if you have a protruding stomach, that poor muscle tone is the main cause; although it's not likely to be the *only* cause. To understand how important strong muscles are to a flat stomach, you have to know a little about what's underneath that flabby exterior.

Inside your stomach are various organs — the largest of which are the intestines. These are literally held *up* by your pelvic girdle — the large part that includes your pubic bone and your seat bones

— and *in* by nothing more than your abdominal muscles and your skin. The abdominals run up and down your stomach as well as criss-crossing it and linking with muscles on your hips, thighs, ribcage and back.

In everyday life, most of our major muscles are used, quite naturally, a reasonable amount just to enable us to carry out what we want to do — our legs have to carry us around, for instance, and our arms have to carry shopping or children. But our stomach muscles — especially if we're sedentary for a long part of the day — don't get used much at all. And so they get out of shape and become slack. And when we *could* use them more, we don't. Sitting down in a chair for instance, your stomach muscles should come into play — but most of us don't bother; we flop down with the aid of gravity and our knees and nothing else.

Muscles need regular work to stay well toned, and because our stomach muscles have to support all those organs, they should really get *more* work, not less. With the right amount of work, even the slackest stomach muscles can be strengthened and shortened. They have tremendous elasticity — which is why after pregnancy women can and do get their flat stomachs back.

Many of you will now be dying to tell me that you have *already* tried intensive stomach exercises — and that they haven't worked.

I do believe you. Interestingly enough, you

could do 100 classic sit-ups a day and they would probably not give you a perfect belly ... though they might give you backache, and they would also help strengthen some of the muscles in your body that don't necessarily *need* strengthening!

Sit-ups only exercise *some* of the stomach muscles — mostly the upper section of the 'rectus abdominus', the vertical, central panel. That's why you won't even *find* a classic sit-up in my programme — there are much BETTER stomach exercises around. Talking of which, maybe you have already flicked through this book and seen one or two exercises that you think you've seen, or tried, before. It could be that you have — but I can bet you have never tried my unique *combination* of exercises, and I can bet even more that you have not learnt *how* to do the exercises. How, as you will find out later, is just as important as what.

With the right system — and that doesn't mean it has to be a lengthy, time-consuming system — you can regain a perfect, strong set of stomach muscles that will not just flatten your stomach but also give you a good waistline. And, as a bonus, when you have strong stomach muscles your whole body should feel better too. Which brings me on to ...

3. IS IT YOUR POSTURE?

This is likely to be either a contributory or a major factor. People with protruding bellies almost always have a posture problem. In fact, very few people have a perfect posture.

The ideal is to be able to stand naturally and send a vertical line through your ear, point of shoulder, hipbone and ankle. (The spine has a natural curve so nobody should try to walk around ramrod-stiff and straight, however.) But many people stand and walk with a 'sway-back' — an exaggerated curve in the small of the back. This automatically makes the pelvic floor tip forward (the back of the pelvis lifts UP and the front moves DOWN) and the stomach, through no fault of its own, sticks out. If this posture is adopted as a daily habit, before long the muscles of the lower back shorten and the stomach muscles lengthen (become weaker), compounding the problem.

If you then decide you want to correct your posture, you have to have not only the will to do so, but also the right exercises to get the muscles back into the right shape.

Bad posture really can become a vicious circle — the weaker your stomach muscles get, the less help they can give to your back to keep the pelvis from tilting and the worse the sway-back becomes. So if your lower back frequently gives you trouble and your stomach looks in poor shape

— suspect bad posture as a prime cause.

The fifteen-day programme will set you on the way to good posture and as your posture improves, your back and your stomach, together, will improve. Your stomach and back get stronger and help your posture; your posture gets better and helps your stomach and back. That's what's called working together!

4. IS IT YOUR DIET?

If your stomach feels taut, uncomfortable or bloated rather than soft or flabby, what and how you eat could be contributing to the problem.

Firstly, certain types of food cause us to retain extra fluid within the body cells. In women, especially, this extra fluid tends to accumulate round the abdomen. For many women, this problem becomes even worse in the seven-ten days before a period and during its first few days — meaning that for up to two weeks out of every month, fluid retention is a real problem.

There's an easy way to tell if you do suffer from fluid retention. If you need to 'go to the loo' infrequently, although you drink normal quantities — you probably do suffer. Your breasts and to a lesser extent your ankles may also swell if this is your problem.

Both PMT and other types of fluid retention

can be minimised with the right diet.

Secondly, the wrong diet may be upsetting your digestive system and causing unacceptable amounts of gas to be produced. Many people complain that their stomachs blow up 'like a balloon' especially after meals. Gas is a natural by-product of the process of food digestion, but many foods, and the way you eat, can cause excessive production — and that blown-up stomach.

Also some people get blown out with air in their bellies — taken in when they swallow.

Lastly, you can never have a completely flat stomach if you suffer from constipation. You need to be regular. The exercise programme will help a great deal by improving the tone of the muscles that help keep you regular — but what, and how, you eat is even more vital.

The Flat Stomach Programme takes all the diet factors into account. With the help of my unique 'Positive/Neutral/Negative' foods guide and a fifteen-day at-a-glance diet plan, you can beat your own particular problems.

To sum up:
- Your unsatisfactory stomach is probably caused by more than one factor.
- Your stomach is not a hopeless case.
- The Flat Stomach Programme will get you there.
    Now, let's take a close look at your DIET …

CHAPTER TWO

The Power of Positive Foods

EATING FOR A FLAT STOMACH

What kind of diet have *you* been eating lately?

Perhaps you've been busy and not paying much attention to food — a quick burger here, a ham sandwich there. Canned beans on toast, plenty of cola, tea and coffee with a few chocolate bars to fill in the gaps.

Or maybe you are the complete opposite; a person who prides himself on healthy eating — lots of wholefoods, muesli, pasta, rice, baked potatoes and pulses.

You'll be interested to know that *either* way, your diet is almost certainly contributing to your stomach problem.

In the last chapter, I explained that a big stomach isn't just caused by lack of exercise. What and how you eat can, and does, contribute to fluid retention, over-production of gas and wind, and constipation. *How much* these problems contribute to the size of your stomach varies tremendously from person to person, but I do believe diet is an important factor for the majority of us.

And by following the Flat Stomach Diet philosophy you can easily minimise the likelihood that your diet is contributing to the shape that you hate!

On the Flat Stomach Diet you will follow the Positive/Neutral/Negative principle.

This means, simply, that you eat plenty of POSITIVE foods — the ones that can actually help dispel the dietary causes of your problem stomach.

Then you eat what you like from the NEUTRAL foods — the ones that have no positive action but which don't add to your problems, either.

Lastly you avoid, as far as possible, the NEGATIVE foods — the ones that, after careful research, I have discovered to be most likely to contribute towards making your stomach unsightly.

For a really flat stomach, you need to take a sideways look at 'healthy eating'. The Flat Stomach Diet teaches you to eat healthily — but in a way that is right for you.

Let's examine again in more detail those 'fat stomach' problems and see how closely they relate to what you eat.

FLUID RETENTION

If you are in good health, the amount of fluid retained in your body is, largely, controllable by *you*.

Although some people naturally retain more than others — and most women will find that they retain much more fluid than usual pre-period and when pregnant — what you eat is the main factor controlling the amount of fluid in your body.

Everybody needs body fluid to survive. The fluid — composed mainly of water and salt — bathes all our cells. Without enough of this fluid they can't work — or live. That is called dehydration. But *more* than enough fluid is pointless, which is why it is perfectly safe to use your diet to cut down on extra fluid. In some circumstances it is actually beneficial to your health; for instance, many women find pre-menstrual stress virtually disappears when they follow a diuretic (fluid elimination) diet.

If you do suffer from surplus fluid, it often accumulates around the stomach area. The difference between a fluid *retaining* diet and a *diuretic* diet can often be several pounds in weight on — or off — your stomach.

So how to achieve a diuretic diet?

The 'culprit' foods are starches and salt.

The starch connection

Foods with the highest concentration of starch are the cereals — bread and breakfast cereals, for instance. Potatoes contain a lot, and so do pulses and, to a lesser extent, some other root vegetables.

Starches are part of the carbohydrate family

that includes fruit, vegetables and sugar. But starches differ from the other types of carbo-hydrate (and from our other sources of energy, fats and protein) in that they require a great deal of water in order to be metabolised within our bodies. They literally have to 'soak up' vast quanti-ties of water as they go through our digestive system — water which otherwise would quickly pass through the system and out of the body.

We all need a certain amount of carbo-hydrates in our diet — around fifty per cent of our total calories should be provided by them. But the way to minimise fluid retention and get enough of the important carbohydrates is to alter the balance of the type of carbohydrates that you eat. You can stay very healthy on a diet that consists of *more* of the low-starch fruits and vegetables and *less* of the cereal and high-starch foods.

I don't recommend that you cut high-starch foods from your diet altogether, but you should avoid the refined ones — white bread, products containing white flour, white pasta, cakes and biscuits, for instance. These refined cereal starches not only contribute *most* to fluid retention but they also offer *least* in nutritional terms. What starch you do eat should come most often from the root vegetables and pulses, then you can include a moderate amount of the unrefined cereals such as wholegrain bread, rice and pasta. These foods *will* cause your body to retain a certain amount of fluid, but because they provide valuable nutrients — and some fibre — they could by no stretch of the imagination be called 'negative' foods.

They are NEUTRAL foods that can, and should, be eaten on the Flat Stomach Diet — but eaten in moderation, especially because, as you will see in a minute, they can also contribute to your fat stomach in another way.

Remember: a high-starch diet (especially refined, white starches) can cause you to retain pints of extra fluid which tends to accumulate around your stomach and may weigh up to 5 lbs (2.5 kgs) (even more for men). A high-starch diet can make your stomach swell up quite alarmingly.

If you think about the last time you went out for a slap-up meal after not eating all that much for a few days, you'll see what I mean. You had a roll while you were ordering, a prawn cocktail with bread and butter; then a pasta main course. By this time you had to loosen your waistband and were wishing you hadn't worn that tight skirt or trousers. You had some gateau for dessert for good measure.

When you stepped on the scales soon afterwards, you'd put on *half a stone* — and your stomach looked five months pregnant. That weight and that bulge were because you just ate a high-starch meal. There is no way the extra weight could be fat — even adding up all the calories you consumed they would only convert to, at most, half a pound or so of fat.

If you go back to your lower-starch diet tomorrow the fluid will quite quickly be eliminated in extra visits to the loo. But if you carry on with this type of diet, you will permanently have that surplus weight around your stomach.

It is fluid, too, that makes every dieter who had just reached target weight and begins to eat normally again, despair after a day of 'normal' eating — she puts on 3 lbs or so and feels she must stay on a low-calorie diet for life. Not true. On the Flat Stomach Diet you can eat plenty of calories — the right sort of calories, though.

The salt connection

Do you like Chinese food? Cream crackers? Ready-salted crisps? Salted peanuts?

If the answer is 'yes', then you are probably a salt-lover, and your addiction could be contributing to fluid retention.

We all need a little salt — about 3 g a day normally. This salt is mostly stored in our body fluid and the amount is carefully monitored. If we don't have enough to drink, or we have been sweating a lot, the salt concentration gets too high and our kidneys excrete less urine to compensate. We also feel thirsty and if we satisfy that thirst, the body's water/salt ratio is restored.

A similar thing happens if we eat a lot of salt — the solution in the body fluids becomes too strong and so we automatically drink more to dilute these levels. If we continue to eat a lot of salt, and we are in perfect health, our kidneys can eliminate the excess salt in our urine. But few of us have perfect kidneys — sluggish circulation, a poor lymph system and recent illness such as flu may all mean that your kidneys aren't working as efficiently as they should, and your body simply retains more fluid to compensate for the extra salt.

At certain times, we all need extra salt — in very hot weather, when we've been doing hard physical work, for instance. But for most of us it is a good idea to cut down on the amount of salt we eat. One way to do this is to stop using salt at the table, another is to use less in cooking. On the Flat Stomach Diet you'll do both of these. But there is also a lot of 'hidden' salt in foods that we eat. Many of the high-starch foods you'll be cutting down on (refined breakfast cereals, for instance) are also often high in salt, so by cutting them down or out you will also be reducing your salt intake. The other high-salt foods are listed at the end of the chapter under NEGATIVE foods.

You can do more to help your body get rid of its excess fluid efficiently than just cut down on starch and salt. You can also eat the foods and drink the liquids that act as natural diuretics. These foods, such as celery and melon, are listed in detail at the end of the chapter under POSITIVE foods, and should be eaten freely.

POOR DIGESTION

If your stomach feels firm or uncomfortable as well as 'blown up', you could be suffering from over-production of gas in your intestines. We all suffer from this at certain times, but some people seem more prone to digestive trouble than others. One thing is for certain — if you want to wear that slinky straight dress or your new swimsuit, you can bet that is the very day your stomach blows up and spoils the whole picture!

Not everyone reacts in the same way to the same foods, either — although certain foods are more *likely* to be the culprits. For instance, kidney and baked beans, certain fruits and onions are some of the most common causes of gas.

For the purposes of the Flat Stomach Diet, I have tried to be sensible when compiling my list of NEGATIVE foods that are likely to cause a gas/wind problem. Obviously if I had tried to include every food that has ever given anyone a problem I would have had to include almost every food. So the list that appears under the NEGATIVE section at the end of the chapter refers to the foods known to me to cause trouble most frequently. I have also starred a few other items in the POSITIVE and NEUTRAL lists which *may* cause a problem for some of you and are therefore best avoided by those people.

How you prepare, cook and eat foods can

also affect whether or not your body has a problem digesting them. The following guidelines will help ensure that whatever foods you eat cause minimal problems.

- Undercooked starches are a common cause of gas in the intestines. Make sure that all bread, pulses, foods containing flour, and potatoes are well cooked.
- Raw vegetables may cause trouble when their cooked counterparts don't. For instance, many people can eat cooked white and red cabbage, but not raw. People who find raw onions a problem may be able to take them in a casserole or soup.
- Very *fresh* bread is likely to cause wind. Eat it slightly stale.
- Any product with yeast in it may cause a problem.
- Some people can't eat wheat products but can eat other grains — rye, oats or rice, all of which can be obtained as bread or low-salt crackers.
- Puréed vegetables and pulses are much easier to digest than whole items. For example, if lentils cause you a problem try puréed lentils in a soup. If the raw oats in muesli don't agree with you, try porridge instead.
- Chop foods small before eating and chew food thoroughly before swallowing.
- Eat little and often — it stands to reason that

your system would prefer to cope with small amounts of food at a time rather than having nothing much to do all day then suddenly receiving a huge meal!

- Eat slowly.

A big factor in indigestion is your own personality — nervous types and people under stress often suffer from a blown-up stomach and other digestive problems. If that sounds like you, add the following tips to the list above:

- Always practise conscious relaxation before you begin to eat. Take a few minutes to breathe slowly and deeply; relax into your chair; let your jaw drop; think about something pleasant.
- Never eat while rushing about and never eat while working or talking on the phone.
- Never try to hurry a meal. However busy you are, you owe it to yourself to have at least a half-hour break for a light or packed lunch; an hour for your evening meal.
- Savour what you are eating. Keep your mouth shut — many people unconsciously gulp in air when they eat. This is a common cause of wind and is frequently a problem with people who eat under stress.

There are a few foods that can actually help

minimise poor digestion in a positive way. These appear in the POSITIVE section at the end of the chapter. I'd recommend the herbal teas, in particular, as an effective antidote.

Because my list of gas- and wind-producing foods has to be subjective, as I said earlier, you may find there are foods on the NEGATIVE list that you can eat perfectly well with no trouble. I have starred these NEGATIVE foods. Any food in the NEGATIVE section with a star by it, you may add to your diet if it causes you no problem. If you are not sure, here is an elimination method that can help you find out:

Have a meal containing nothing but the POSITIVE foods plus a small portion of NEUTRAL protein food. To this meal, add an average portion of your chosen NEGATIVE food. At your next meal, make sure to eat only POSITIVE and NEUTRAL foods. If, when a six-hour period is up, you have experienced no adverse reaction to the NEGATIVE food, you can add it to your diet as a NEUTRAL. Don't test more than one NEGATIVE food at a time, otherwise, if you do get a bad reaction, you won't know which one caused it.

CONSTIPATION

Ironically, many of the foods that are known to trigger over-production of gas in the intestines (such as whole grains, pulses and certain dried fruits) are also the very ones most frequently recommended by doctors and dieticians as a cure for, or the prevention of, constipation.

And certainly you need a regular bowel movement for a really flat stomach. But there is no point in preventing constipation with a high cereal, pulse and dried fruit-fibre diet if all you do is blow your stomach up with uncomfortable wind instead.

We have to replace a diet high in those foods with a diet that is equally good at preventing constipation but without that unwanted side-effect. This is easily done by increasing the amount of fruit and legumes in your diet. Citrus fruits and all the lovely summer fruits such as berries and plums are ideal. Melons are wonderful because they not only have a good fibre content, but they are also a diuretic. In fact all fruit helps fluid elimination, making it doubly perfect for the Flat Stomach Diet.

Add to that all the legumes — whole green beans, peas, corn kernels, and salads as well as certain types of dried fruit, and you have a delicious diet that is very high in fibre.

But it isn't *just* fibre that keeps you regular. I believe that more constipation is caused by not drinking enough water or eating enough citrus fruit than ever was caused by not getting enough bran in your diet!

You absolutely MUST drink a lot of water on the Flat Stomach Diet. At least three pints a day for preference. Drinking a lot of water will not cause fluid retention, I can assure you. The surplus will simply be flushed immediately out of your system but all that water will keep you regular, as well as improving the condition of your skin, gums and eyes. Yes, you will have to go to the toilet frequently — but that's a small price to pay for a flat stomach and good health, isn't it?

Citrus fruits, particularly oranges, seem to work to cure constipation in people for whom every other method (including tons of bran and laxatives) has failed. I don't know why it works, but it does.

Lastly, the Flat Stomach exercise regime will help prevent constipation by strengthening the internal muscles that control the bowels and digestive system and therefore making them more efficient.

To sum up — you will have regular bowels if you eat enough of the POSITIVE foods, particularly citrus fruits, if you eat moderate amounts of the NEUTRAL unrefined starch foods, drink plenty of water and take regular exercise, including the Flat Stomach regime.

A complete list of POSITIVE, NEUTRAL and NEGATIVE foods appears at the end of this chapter.

A word of caution: if you don't suffer from constipation, over-indulgence in citrus and other fruits may result in a loose bowel. If that happens, cut down the amount accordingly until you find your own level.

DESIGNING YOUR OWN DIET

On the pages that follow, you will find a comprehensive list of all the POSITIVE/NEUTRAL/NEGATIVE foods we've been discussing.

The fifteen-day Flat Stomach Diet in Chapter 3 is built on the P-N-N theory and has been thoroughly tested by me. You need do no more than follow it as it stands and see almost instant results in your slimmer silhouette over the next fifteen days.

However, you may have particular likes and dislikes, or you may want to add more variety to your diet so you can continue eating in this new way after the fifteen days are up. You can build a diet to suit yourself — one which you can stay on for the rest of your life — very easily. In fact, it couldn't be easier!

All you do is choose as many items as you can every day from the POSITIVE list. Try to include one or two at every meal — or, in the case of drinks, with every meal.

Make up the rest of your diet from the NEUTRAL foods, getting as wide a variety as you can, bearing in mind that over-indulgence in the unrefined starches will lead to a certain amount of fluid retention — some people are more prone to this than others.

The NEGATIVE list contains the foods that you should avoid as far as possible (with the exception of any starred items which you can include in your diet if they have passed the elimination test described on page 26).

Weight maintenance

Because the POSITIVE foods tend to be low in calories and the NEGATIVE foods tend to be high in calories, most people should find no problem maintaining their weight on the regime. It is most unlikely that anyone would put *on* weight following the POSITIVE/NEUTRAL/NEGATIVE theory.

If you find you are losing weight on the diet but don't want to, or if you want to put on weight, simply add more of the high-oil NEUTRAL foods to your diet and a few more of the unrefined starches.

Weight loss

If you follow the regime properly you don't need to count calories — simply eat more fruits, vegetables and NEUTRAL proteins and you should lose weight slowly. For further help, consult the calorie chart at the back of the book.

As an approximate guide to how many calories you should be eating, most men will maintain their weight on approximately 2,750 calories a day and will lose weight on 1,500-1,750 calories a day. Most women will maintain their weight on about 2,000 calories a day and will lose weight on 1,000-1,250 calories a day.

Don't forget that when you begin the Flat Stomach Diet, most of you will lose at least a few pounds in weight which is *fluid* loss, not fat. If you then follow the 1,250-calorie fifteen-day diet, you will continue to lose weight. If you follow the Maintenance fifteen-day diet, your weight should stabilise after day three.

POSITIVE FOODS

Eat freely from all these foods.

To help eliminate fluid
ALL fresh fruit, especially:

Watermelon	Strawberries
All other types of melon	Raspberries
Citrus fruits	Pineapple
Peaches	Cherries
Nectarines	

The juice of these fruits

Salad vegetables:

Celery	Lettuce
Tomatoes	Watercress
Sweet peppers	Cucumber
Fennel	

The juice of these salad vegetables

The following herbs, fresh, chopped:
Parsley
Sweet cicely
Lovage

Grated horseradish root
To drink:
> Mineral water, water, water with lemon juice
> added
> Dandelion tea
> All fruit teas, especially orange and lemon

To reduce digestive problems and gas
Live natural yogurt
Peppermint tea
Chamomile tea
Lemon balm tea
Fresh ginger
The following, fresh, chopped:

Sage	Fennel leaves
Basil	Dill leaves
Marjoram	

Seeds of:
> Fennel
> Anise
> Dill

For bowel regularity
All fresh fruit, especially oranges and other citrus
fruit

Raspberries	Rhubarb*
Blackberries	Gooseberries*
Blackcurrants	Kiwifruit
Apricots	Bananas
Plums	Grapes
Cherries	

The following fresh or frozen vegetables:

Peas*	Spinach
Sweetcorn	Broad beans*
Baby corn kernels	Mushrooms
Mangetout	Asparagus
Whole beans	Spring greens
Leeks	Kale
Broccoli	Primo cabbage
Cauliflower	Carrots
Runner beans	Swede
Aubergine	Turnip
Brussels sprouts*	

Saladstuff:

Beansprouts	Tomatoes
Mushrooms	Raw cauliflower
Celery	Raw carrots
Sweet peppers	Cress

Miscellaneous: Hot chilli, ground

Dried fruits:
    Dried apricots
    Dried peaches
    Dried dates
    Dried figs*

To drink: Orange juice, preferably fresh
    mineral water, water

* These foods may cause a gas problem in a
    minority of people. If so, avoid.

NOTE: The NEUTRAL starches will also help a
regular bowel.

NEUTRAL FOODS

Proteins
All poultry
All fish, fresh or frozen, except shrimps/prawns
Tuna, mackerel, sardines, salmon, in oil, well
    drained, moderate portions only
Eggs
Lean beef
Veal
Lean fillet of lamb
Liver, kidneys
Game: wild duck, pheasant, grouse, partridge,
    rabbit
Fresh shelled nuts*
Peanut butter
Tofu
Sunflower seeds
Cottage cheese
Skimmed milk soft cheese
Half-fat soft cheese
Fromage frais
Brie, Camembert, Edam, Boursin, Bel Paese,
    Mozzarella, Parmesan, Gruyère — all
    moderate portions only
Yogurt
Skimmed and semi-skimmed milk

Carbohydrates
Artichokes, globe and Jerusalem
Beetroot

Radish
Mustard and cress
Avocado
Onion, well boiled, baked or casseroled
Fruit tinned in natural juice
Vegetables, canned, drained and reheated in water
     not brine
Squash/marrow
Courgettes

Restricted starches
(Moderate portions, maximum three times a day for
women, four times a day for men from this group)
Wholewheat bread, well cooked
Rye bread
Oatbran bread
Rice crackers, low-salt
Rye crispbreads, low-salt
Oatcakes
Wholewheat pasta
Wholegrain rice, wild rice
Wheatgerm bread, e.g. Hovis
Wholewheat pitta
Potatoes, boiled, baked
Sweet potato
Lentils, brown or green, well cooked and puréed*
Porridge
Low-salt wholegrain breakfast cereals: 'no added
     salt' muesli, Shredded Wheat, Weetabix

Miscellaneous
Sugar (restrict to occasional use), honey, reduced
    sugar fruit spreads
Oils of all kinds
Butter (use sparingly)
Vegetable margarines, low-fat spread
Apple juice
Vinegar
Fresh herbs, other than those already listed
Dried herbs and spices
Non-dairy cream (e.g. Elmlea)
Mayonnaise
Cornflour (use sparingly)
Wine and other alcohol (occasional use)
Garlic/purée*
Soya sauce (use sparingly)
Worcestershire sauce (use sparingly)
French dressing
Oyster sauce
* These foods may cause a gas problem in a
  minority of people. If so, avoid.

NEGATIVE FOODS

*Refined starch foods — avoid to minimise fluid
retention*
White bread
White rice
Sweet biscuits

Cream crackers
Cakes, particularly sponges
Gateau
Scones
Crumpets
Doughnuts
Milk puddings, e.g. rice pudding, tapioca
Pastries
Fruit pies
Meat pies and pasties
White pastry
White sauce
Refined breakfast cereals, e.g. Rice Krispies, Corn-
    flakes
Trifles, packet pudding mixes

High salt foods
Yeast extract
Gammon
Bacon
Smoked haddock
Kippers
Smoked mackerel, smoked trout
Smoked salmon
Smoked cheese
Ham
Olives
Salami and other deli sausages
Black pudding
Shrimps, prawns
Cheddar cheese

Blue cheese
Processed cheese slices
Pickle
Monosodium glutamate
Corned beef
Crisps
Cornflakes
All Bran
Cream crackers
Tinned and packet soups
Ketchup
Luncheon meat
Canned beans
Canned spaghetti
Gravy mix
And, of course, cooking salt and table salt, including sea salt.

Foods that may upset digestion/increase gases
NOTE: People's tolerance towards these foods varies greatly. If a food is marked with a * and you would particularly like to include it in your diet, try the elimination test on page 26. If it passes, you can then add it to your NEUTRAL list.
Animal fats — lard, dripping, suet
All deep-fried foods
Whole milk*
Cream, single* cream, soured* cream, double cream, non-dairy*
Pastry, white
Pastry, wholemeal

Colas and fizzy drinks
Tea*
Coffee*
Chocolate
Shoulder of lamb and any fatty cuts of red meat
Farmed duck
Goose
Pork, lean*
Pork, crackling
Highly spiced foods — e.g. Madras curry*
Stout*, beer*, lager*
Granary bread* (add to restricted starches)
Bran
Raw white and red cabbage*
Raw onion*, fried onion
Chick peas* (add to restricted starches)
Kidney beans* (add to restricted starches)
Baked beans, reduced salt* (add to restricted
      starches)
Soya protein (meat substitute) and soya beans*
Sultanas*, currants*, raisins*, prunes*
Mincemeat

CHAPTER THREE

The Fifteen-Day Flat Stomach Diet

Eating for a flat stomach really is easy when you know how! You can devise your own diet from the information in Chapter 2 if you like — but, to make things easy, I've planned out a tasty yet simple fifteen-day diet for you to follow while you complete the Exercise Programme. Because of its flexibility, it's suitable for dieters and non-dieters alike.

You eat FIVE times a day — a light breakfast, two portable snacks, and two larger meals — a lunch and an evening meal. If it suits you better, you can swop these two around and have your main meal at lunchtime. However, the lunch can be packed to take to work — all you need is a lunchbox and a couple of lidded plastic containers, plus some foil or cling-film. A vacuum flask would also be handy.

The basic diet is straightforward and all the meals are easy to prepare. That doesn't mean they're boring — far from it. In addition, for keener cooks, I've devised some recipes as alternatives to some of the meals. There is one every day and you'll find them all in Chapter 4.

Before beginning the diet, you must read the following notes.

IF YOU WANT TO LOSE WEIGHT

The basic diet averages around 1,200 calories a day, which is ideal for women wanting to lose 5-7 lbs (2.3-3.2 kgs) in the fifteen days. If you want to follow this slimming diet, just eat and drink all the foods and drinks listed EXCEPT THOSE IN ITALICS IN THE BRACKETS. If two amounts follow a food (e.g. 4 oz/100 g (*6 oz/175 g*) potato), you eat the first amount, in this case 4 oz/100 g. If extra items appear in bracketed italics (e.g. the dessert after the main meal on Day 1 reads, '8 oz/ 225 g slice melon (*plus 3 oz/75 g vanilla ice-cream*)', you just eat the melon.

IF YOU WANT A MAINTENANCE DIET

The Maintenance Diet is higher in calories and is suitable for women wishing to maintain their weight. To follow the Maintenance Diet, all you do is eat everything listed, including the amounts/ items shown in italics in brackets. For instance, if a meal includes 4 oz/100 g (*6 oz/175 g*) potato, you eat 6 oz/175 g. If complete extra items are listed (e.g. on Day 1, dessert after the main meal is 8 oz/

225g slice melon (*plus 3oz/75g vanilla ice-cream*)), you eat the melon and the ice-cream. If the item in brackets begins with the word 'or', you eat that item *instead* of the preceding item.

FOR MEN

If you are male and want to lose weight, you can follow the Maintenance Diet as described above which should help you to lose around 5-7 lbs (2.3-3.2 kgs) in the fifteen days. If you don't want to lose weight, turn to Chapter 9 for more diet information.

DRINKS

Everyone has a daily skimmed milk allowance of ¼ pint/150 ml (basic) or ½ pint/300 ml (maintenance). You can use this to have with tea or coffee if you are including either of those on your diet (they are optional). If you stick to fruit and herbal teas and other drinks, you should have the milk allowance as a drink on its own — before bedtime would be a good idea.

Some additional drinks are mentioned within the diet. Fruit juices, for instance, are quite high in calories and should only be drunk when specified. Herbal and fruit teas are virtually calorie-free and you can drink as much of them as you like. Twinings and Secret Garden are two brands I enjoy. You must drink plenty of water — I suggest six glasses a day, spaced out evenly throughout the day.

SALT

The diet is low in salt. I've suggested using a salt substitute (such as Ruthmol or LoSalt) in some of the dishes if you find them too bland. Salt substitute is optional throughout. Or you could cut down the amount of salt you use gradually and you'll soon find you need hardly any. Just use your common sense.

Packet gravies are high in salt — make your own using the cooking juices with a little vegetable or chicken stock and/or a little white or red wine, depending on the dish. You can thicken it with one teaspoon cornflour — about the only refined starch you'll find on this diet!

VEGETARIANS AND NON-MEAT EATERS

Although I have included red meat, poultry and fish on the diet because the vast majority of people still enjoy meat, you can still follow the diet whether you're a total vegetarian or simply don't eat red meat. Any necessary substitutes are suggested each day at the end of the day's diet.

UNLIMITEDS

All these are unlimited on the diet: fresh and dried herbs; lemon juice, salad leaves of any kind, herb teas, fruit teas, water, mineral water.

DON'T FORGET!

Lastly, don't forget all the eating tips in the previous chapter — most importantly — eat SLOWLY, relax and enjoy your food.

DAY 1

On rising
Cup lemon tea

Breakfast
5 fl oz/150 ml (*6 fl oz/175 ml*) glass orange juice
5 fl oz/150 ml (*6 fl oz/175 ml*) bowl Greek strained yogurt
1 banana chopped in

Snack
1 rye crispbread spread with 2 oz/50 g cottage cheese

Lunch
2 oz/50 g (*3 oz/75 g*) Brie
2 rye crispbreads with low-fat spread
Mixed salad of tomato, lettuce (any type), watercress, red pepper, cucumber and chopped basil tossed in oil-free French dressing
1 peach or apple

Snack
²/₃ oz/15 g (*1 oz/25 g*) sunflower seeds
Cup herb tea

Main Meal
Medium (*large*) portion grilled, baked or microwaved chicken
3 oz/75 g (*5 oz/150 g*) new potatoes
Salad of 1 stick celery, chopped, ½ apple, ½ oz/ 12 g walnuts, all mixed in 1 dessertspoon reduced-calorie mayonnaise and 1 dessertspoon natural yogurt plus 1 teaspoon lemon juice, chopped parsley
OR
1 portion Saffron Chicken with Orange Rice (see recipe page 68)
OR
1 portion Honeyed Chicken (see recipe page 70)

plus 5 tablespoons brown rice
8 oz/225 g slice melon (*plus 3 oz/75 g vanilla ice-cream*) with any selection

Vegetarian suggestion: small baked potato filled with portion dahl (lentil purée) with celery and apple side salad.

DAY 2

On rising
Fruit tea, any variety

Breakfast
A mixed fresh fruit salad of melon, strawberries or kiwifruit, pineapple, apple and banana — total approx 10 oz/275 g
2 oz/50 g (*4 oz/100 g*) natural fromage frais
1 teaspoon honey

Snack
2 rice cakes spread with 1 dessertspoon (*1 tablespoon*) peanut butter

Lunch
Salad as Day 1
½ a small (*medium*) ripe avocado filled with oil-free French dressing (*or filled with traditional French dressing*)

1 small (*medium*) slice wholemeal bread with low-fat spread

Snack
1 fruit yogurt
(*plus 1¹/₂oz/35g dried 'no need to soak' apricots*)

Main Meal
6oz/175g (*8oz/225g*) fillet white fish, any variety, baked, grilled or microwaved
4oz/100g (*6oz/175g*) jacket potato
(*¹/₂oz/15g butter*)
5oz/150g (*6oz/175g*) broccoli and 3oz/75g (*4oz/100g*) whole beans, lightly cooked
Lemon juice garnish
OR
1 portion Italian Fish Steaks (see recipe on page 70) plus 3oz/75g (*5oz/150g*) new potatoes and 4oz/100g (*5oz/150g*) broccoli
OR
1 portion Sole in Mushroom Sauce (see recipe page 71) plus 4oz/100g (*6oz/175g*) new potatoes and 3oz/75g (*4oz/100g*) French beans
1 orange and 1 kiwifruit with any selection

Vegetarian suggestion: add 1oz/25g flaked toasted almonds to the vegetables before serving. Add 1 small serving Brie to the fruit dessert.

DAY 3

On rising
Lemon tea

Breakfast
1/2 (*whole*) grapefruit
1 1/2 oz/35 g (*2 1/2 oz/65 g*) 'no added salt' muesli
with 4 fl oz/100 ml (*5 fl oz/150 ml*) skimmed milk

Snack
2 oz/50 g skimmed milk soft cheese or cottage
cheese
1 stick celery and 2 dates

Lunch
1 (*2*) hard-boiled egg/s, halved on bed of lettuce
and covered with 1 (*1 1/2*) tablespoon/s reduced-
calorie mayonnaise
Watercress or parsley to garnish
1 small (*medium*) slice wholemeal bread with low-
fat spread
1 orange

Snack
1 oz/25 g (*2 oz/50 g*) shelled hazelnuts
5 fl oz natural low-fat yogurt

Main Meal
1 medium (*large*) extra-lean trimmed lamb chop,
grilled

4 oz/100 g peas, fresh or frozen, or mangetout
4 oz/100 g (*6 oz/175 g*) carrots or leeks, lightly cooked
3 oz/75 g (*4 oz/100 g*) low-salt instant mashed potato
2 teaspoons mint sauce
OR
1 portion Moroccan Lamb (see recipe on page 72) with 3 (*5*) tablespoons boiled brown rice
OR
1 portion Braised Citrus Beef (see recipe page 73) plus large portion spring greens and 3 oz/75 g (*4 oz/100 g*) new potatoes
4 oz/100 g cherries or 1 apple with any selection

Vegetarian suggestion: serve 1 × 4 oz/100 g Vege-Burger instead of the lamb or beef
OR
have 1 portion Nutty Red Peppers (see recipe page 79)

DAY 4

On rising
4 fl oz/100 ml (*5 fl oz/150 ml*) glass orange juice

Breakfast
2 oz/150 g 'no need to soak' dried apricots, chopped and stirred into 4 oz/100 g (*5 oz/150 g*) Greek strained yogurt

Snack
1 apple
1 rice cake topped with 2oz/50g skimmed milk, soft cheese and cucumber

Lunch
8oz/225g slice melon
3oz/75g (*4oz/100g*) cooked chicken
Cucumber and tomato salad with chopped basil
1 small wholemeal roll with low-fat spread (*or 1/4oz/10g butter*)
OR
1 portion of Chicken, Rice and Beansprout salad (see recipe page 73)

Snack
1 orange
(*plus 1oz/25g sunflower seeds*)

Main Meal
1/2 grapefruit
4oz/100g (*5oz/150g*) salmon steak or 6oz/175g (*8oz/225g*) trout, poached or baked or microwaved
4oz/100g mangetout
3oz/75g (*6oz/175g*) new potatoes with 1/4oz/10g butter
Lemon juice and wedges to garnish
OR
1 portion Fennel Trout (see recipe page 74) with

3 oz/75 g (*4oz/100g*) new potatoes tossed in low-fat spread plus 3 oz/75 g mangetout
4 oz/100 g strawberries, raspberries or cherries or 1 kiwifruit with either selection

Vegetarian suggestion: use 4 oz/100 g (*5oz/150g*) diced tofu in your lunchtime salad; 1 × 4 oz/100 g (*5oz/150g*) nut cutlet instead of the salmon.

DAY 5

On rising
Lemon tea

Breakfast
1 ½ oz/35 g any wholegrain, low-salt breakfast cereal (e.g. 2 Weetabix, Shreddies) with skimmed milk to cover

Snack
8 oz/225 g slice melon or 1 orange
1 oz/25 g (*2oz/50g*) Edam cheese

Lunch
A salad of 2 oz/50 g (*3oz/75g*) tuna in oil, well drained and mixed with chopped cucumber, celery, apple and 4 oz/100 g (*5oz/150g*) cooked weight wholewheat pasta, all tossed in oil-free French

dressing and served on a bed of salad leaves and garnished with chopped parsley

Snack
Slice melon
1 Petit Fromage Frais with Fruit

Main Meal
1 medium (*large*) breast of chicken portion, skinned and covered with a paste of 2 fl oz/50 ml natural low-fat yogurt mixed with 1 dessertspoon tandoori powder and grilled over medium heat for 30 minutes or baked for 45 minutes
3 oz/75 g (*6 oz/175 g*) boiled wholegrain rice
2 tablespoons chopped cucumber and natural yogurt
1 tomato, sliced and garnished with chopped basil
OR
1 portion Chicken Paprika (see recipe on page 75)
OR
1 portion Sherried Turkey (see recipe on page 76), either choice served with 4 oz/100 g (*5 oz/150 g*) new potatoes and a green side salad with lemon dressing
(*plus 1 glass dry white wine or 2 oz/50 g ice-cream with any selection*)

Vegetarian suggestion: use 2 oz/50 g Mozzarella cheese in the lunchtime salad; have 1 medium baked aubergine in the evening, sprinkled with

1 oz/25 g toasted sesame seeds, plus the rice and side dishes.

DAY 6

On rising
4 fl oz/100 ml (*5 fl oz/150 ml*) orange juice

Breakfast
5 fl oz/150 ml   (*6 fl oz/175 ml*)   natural   low-fat yogurt topped with 4 oz/100 g (*6 oz/175 g*) straw-berries, raspberries or sliced kiwifruit plus ½ oz/15 g oatflakes

Snack
1 (*2*) rye crispbreads spread with 1 dessertspoon (*1 tablespoon*) peanut butter

Lunch
Slice melon
A salad of 2 oz/50 g (*2½ oz/65 g*) hazelnuts or unsalted peanuts mixed with 6 oz/175 ml carrot, grated and 1 oz/25 g dates, chopped plus 1 teaspoon anise seeds (optional), all tossed in a dressing of 1 dessertspoon olive oil mixed with 2 fl oz/50 ml orange juice, pepper and a little salt substitute
1 mini pitta or ½ pitta

Snack
1 orange and 1 banana

Main Meal
4 oz/100 g (*5 oz/150 g*) extra lean roast beef
2 oz/50 g (*3 oz/75 g*) new potatoes
4 oz/100 g cauliflower
4 oz/100 g spring greens
4 oz/100 g swede, puréed
1 dessertspoon home-made horseradish sauce
Gravy made from beef juices and a little beef stock, thickened with 1 teaspoon cornflour
OR
1 portion Stir-Fried Beef with Oyster Sauce (see recipe page 76)
OR
1 portion Mushroom Pilau (see recipe page 77)

DAY 7

On rising
Fruit tea, any variety

Breakfast
½ a grapefruit
1 boiled egg
1 rye crispbread with low-fat spread
(*or 1 medium slice wholemeal bread with low-fat spread*)

Snack
1 peach or nectarine
1 Petit Fromage Frais (fruit variety)

Lunch
2 oz/50 g Mozzarella, sliced
2 medium tomatoes, sliced
Chopped basil
1 dessertspoon olive oil
Leaf salad of choice
(*plus 1 medium slice bread with low-fat spread*)

Snack
1 (*2*) rye crispbread/s with 2 oz/50 g (*4 oz/100 g*)
half-fat soft cheese
1 orange

Main Meal
4 oz/100 g (*6 oz/175 g*) lamb's liver or 2 (*3*)
lamb's kidneys, grilled or fried in non-stick pan in
teaspoon corn oil
3 oz/75 g (*4 oz/100 g*) new potatoes
5 oz/150 g broccoli
2 oz/50 g broad beans
1 medium tomato
A gravy made from cooking juices plus 1 fl oz/
25 ml red wine, little water, 1 teaspoon tomato
purée and 1 teaspoon cornflour
OR
1 portion Liver Stir-Fry (see recipe page 78)

served with 4 (*6*) tablespoons boiled brown rice
OR
1 portion Nutty Red Peppers (see recipe page 79)
plus a green salad
2 oz/50 g (*3 oz/75 g*) ice-cream or 1 glass dry
wine with any selection

Vegetarian suggestion: substitute cubed tofu for
the liver in the stir-fry.

DAY 8

On rising
Fruit tea, any variety

Breakfast
5 oz/150 g (*6 oz/175 g*) Greek strained yogurt
with 6 oz/175 g (*8 oz/225 g*) mixed fresh fruit,
chopped, and 1 teaspoon honey

Snack
1 banana
1 oz/25 g (*2 oz/50 g*) dried apricots

Lunch
2 rye crispbreads with low-fat spread
Fruit and cheese salad: combine 2 oz/50 g (*3 oz/
75 g*) cubed Edam cheese with 4 oz/100 g (*5 oz/
150 g*) cubed melon or melon balls, 1 ring fresh (or

canned in natural juice) pineapple, cubed, 2oz/
150g cucumber, diced, and toss in lemon juice
with pinch ground ginger. Garnish with chopped
parsley

Snack
1 orange
1 Petit Fromage Frais with Fruit (*or 1 fruit yogurt*)

Main meal
6oz/175g (*8oz/ 225g*) fillet of monkfish or cod,
baked in foil or microwaved
4oz/100g sliced green peppers and 4oz/100g
sliced tomato, stir-fried in a non-stick pan in 1
dessertspoon corn oil
3oz/75g (*6oz/175g*) boiled wholegrain rice
OR
1 portion Monkfish Kebabs (see recipe page 80)
served with 3 (*5*) tablespoons boiled brown rice
OR
1 portion Tangy Plaice (see recipe page 81) plus
4oz/100g (*5oz/125g*) new potatoes and 3oz/
75g (*5oz/125g*) broccoli

Vegetarian suggestion: par-boil 1 cubed aubergine,
brush with corn oil and use on kebabs instead of
the fish in the recipe on page 80.

DAY 9

On rising
Lemon tea

Breakfast
As Day 1

Snack
1 (*2*) rye crispbread/s
1 stick celery and 2 oz/50 g (*4 oz/100 g*) cottage cheese

Lunch
Salad Niçoise: Combine 1 hard-boiled egg, roughly chopped, with 3 oz/75 g (*4 oz/100 g*) tuna in oil, well drained, 3 oz/75 g (*4 oz/100 g*) cold cooked potato, diced
3 oz/75 g cooked cooled whole green beans, 1 firm tomato, chopped, 4 oz/100 g crisp lettuce, chopped and mixed with oil-free French dressing (*or traditional French dressing*)

Snack
1 orange
1 apple or peach

Main Meal
4 oz/100 g (*6 oz/175 g*) roast chicken, lean only
5 oz/150 g courgettes, sliced, and 1 sliced tomato,

stir-fried in 1 dessertspoon corn oil
3 oz/75 g mangetout
3 oz/75 g (*5 oz/150 g*) sweetcorn
1 teaspoon cornflour to thicken meat juices if liked
OR
1 portion Chicken Satay with Peanut Sauce (see recipe page 82)
OR
1 portion Stuffed Chicken Breasts (see recipe page 83) with 2 oz/50 g (*4 oz/100 g*) sweet potato and a green salad

Vegetarian suggestion: use 2 eggs in the salad and omit the tuna; serve 4 oz/100 g (*6 oz/175 g*) Vege-Burger instead of the chicken.

DAY 10

On rising
Fruit tea, any variety

Breakfast
As Day 2

Snack
2 oz/50 g cottage cheese on 1 stick celery

Lunch
1 small (*medium*) slice wholemeal bread with low-fat spread
Salad of 3oz/75g baby sweetcorn, 4oz/100g tender broad beans and 2oz/50g whole green beans, all lightly cooked and cooled, mixed with ½oz/15g (*1oz/25g*) walnut halves and a dressing of natural low-fat yogurt mixed with 1 dessertspoon reduced-calorie mayonnaise, lemon juice and pinch cayenne pepper

Snack
1 dessertspoon (*1 tablespoon*) peanut butter on 1 (*2*) rye crispbread/s

Main Meal
4oz/150g grilled beefburger made with extra lean fine minced beef, mixed herbs, 1 teaspoon tomato purée and dash Worcestershire sauce
1oz/25g grated Edam cheese, melted on top
4oz/100g (*8oz/225g*) jacket potato
5oz/150g aubergine, stir-fried in 1 dessertspoon oil with teaspoon cumin seed and puréed
OR
1 portion Stuffed Aubergine (see recipe page 83)
OR
1 portion Minty Lamb Kebabs (see recipe page 85) with 6 tablespoons brown rice and a tomato salad

Vegetarian suggestion: for your main meal, have an individual vegetarian wholemeal pizza plus green salad — or, in the recipe, use soya mince instead of the beef or have 1 portion Lentil Bolognese (see recipe page 92).

DAY 11

On rising
Lemon tea

Breakfast
As Day 3

Snack
1 oz/25 g Edam cheese and 1 stick celery

Lunch
12 oz/350 g bowl home-made Lentil Soup (see recipe page 85)
1 orange (*plus 1 banana*)

Snack
1 oz/25 g sunflower seeds

Main Meal
4 oz/100 g (*6 oz/175 g*) lean lamb steak, cooked in foil with 2 oz/50 g sliced red peppers and 1

teaspoon chopped dill
4 oz/100 g mangetout
4 oz/100 g broccoli
OR
1 portion Veal and Aubergine Casserole (see recipe page 86) with 3 oz/75 g cooked-weight brown rice or wholewheat pasta
6 oz/175 g soft fruit of choice plus 1 fl oz/25 ml (*2 fl oz/50 ml*) Elmlea cream substitute or Greek yogurt, with either selection

Vegetarian suggestion: baked $\frac{1}{2}$ ripe avocado sprinkled with lemon juice, instead of the lamb.

DAY 12

On rising
4 fl oz/100 ml (*5 fl oz/150 ml*) orange juice

Breakfast
As Day 4

Snack
1 banana
(*plus $\frac{1}{2}$ oz/15 g sunflower seeds*)

Lunch
$\frac{1}{2}$ small (*medium*) avocado, filled with a mixture of 1 × 43 g tin dressed crab mixed with 1

tablespoon reduced-calorie mayonnaise and 1 teaspoon lemon juice, served on a bed of lettuce and garnished with chopped parsley
(*plus 1 medium slice wholemeal bread*)
Slice melon

Snack
1 punnet strawberries or 1 orange
1 natural fromage frais

Main Meal
2-egg omelette cooked in $\frac{1}{4}$oz/10g ($\frac{1}{2}$oz/15g) butter and filled with 3oz/75g chopped button mushrooms and 2oz/50g sweetcorn
Leaf salad
1 small (*medium*) slice bread with low-fat spread
OR
1 portion Baked Egg Ratatouille (see recipe page 87)
OR
1 portion Courgette Gratin (see recipe page 88)

Vegetarian suggestion: fill the avocado with 2oz/50g cottage cheese mixed with $\frac{1}{2}$oz/15g walnuts or chopped mixed nuts.

DAY 13

On rising
Lemon tea

Breakfast
As Day 5

Snack
1 orange
½oz/15g (*1oz/25g*) sunflower seeds

Lunch
1 portion Salad Soup (see recipe page 88)
2oz/50g Brie and 2 rye crispbreads

Snack
1 nectarine or apple and 2oz/50g (*4oz/100g*) cherries or grapes
(*plus 1 diet fruit yogurt*)

Main Meal
1 medium trout (about 7oz/200g), grilled, micro-waved or fried in non-stick pan in 1 teaspoon corn oil (covered)
1oz/25g (*2oz/50g*) flaked almonds, lightly browned
2oz/50g (*4oz/150g*) new potatoes
3oz/75g (*4oz/100g*) whole beans or chopped spinach
3oz/75g (*4oz/100g*) peas
OR
1 portion Salmon in Lemon Cream (see recipe page 89) plus 4oz/100g (*5oz/125g*) new potatoes and 3oz/75g green beans

Vegetarian suggestion: serve 1 nut cutlet instead of the fish; toss the vegetables in ½oz/15g chopped mixed nuts.

DAY 14

On rising
4 fl oz/100 ml (*5 fl oz/150 ml*) orange juice

Breakfast
As Day 6

Snack
2 rice crackers spread with 1 dessertspoon (*1 tablespoon*) peanut butter

Lunch
Salad of crisp lettuce, chopped celery, sliced red peppers and diced cucumber with 2 oz/50 g Edam cheese
1 rye crispbread with low-fat spread (*or 1 medium slice wholemeal bread with low-fat spread*)

Snack
1 apple
1 Petit Fromage Frais with Fruit

Main Meal
1 medium (*large*) chicken portion spread with a

little garlic purée (optional) and 1 teaspoon crushed rosemary, grilled or baked
3 oz/75 g broad beans
4 oz/100 g carrots or chopped spinach
3 oz/75 g (*6 oz/175 g*) boiled wholegrain rice
OR
1 portion Ginger Chicken (see recipe page 90)
OR
1 portion Liver with Sage (see recipe page 91) with 3 oz/75 g new potatoes and 3 oz/75 g spinach
1 orange
(*plus 2 oz/50 g vanilla ice-cream or 1 glass dry wine with any selection*)

Vegetarian suggestion: instead of the main meal, serve 1 × 5 oz/150 g slice vegetarian wholemeal quiche plus a mixed salad.

DAY 15

On rising
Fruit tea

Breakfast
As Day 7

Snack
1 diet fruit yogurt

1 nectarine or 1 apple
(*plus 1 banana*)

Lunch
Salad of 4 oz/100 g broccoli florets and 2 oz/50 g
mangetout, both lightly cooked, mixed with 2 oz/
50 g diced red pepper, 1 oz/25 g (*2 oz/50 g*)
almonds and a dressing of 1 tablespoon olive oil
mixed with lemon juice and seasoning, served on a
bed of fresh spinach leaves or radicchio
1 orange

Snack
2 oz/50 g cottage cheese
2 rye crispbreads with low-fat spread
(*plus 1 oz/25 g Brie*)

Main Meal
5 oz/150 g (*6 oz/175 g*) steak, trimmed of all fat
and grilled
3 oz/75 g whole beans
2 oz/50 g (*4 oz/100 g*) new potatoes
¼ oz/10 g butter to garnish
OR
1 portion Mustard Steak (see recipe page 91)
served with beans and potato but no butter
OR
1 portion Lentil Bolognese (see recipe page 92)
8 oz/225 g mixed fresh fruit of choice with any
selection

CHAPTER FOUR

Recipes for a Flat Stomach

All these recipes are optional instead of a simpler meal within the fifteen-day diet. All serve two except where stated otherwise; though quantities for most dishes can be doubled to serve four or halved to serve one.

My selections make full use of the POSITIVE foods and show how you can eat tastily and well while keeping that stomach flat!

Saffron Chicken (Day 1)
220 calories per portion

2 medium breast of chicken portions, skin removed

Garlic purée or paste equivalent to 2 cloves

Pinch ground ginger, or tiny knob fresh

½ teaspoon cardamom, ground

Pinch chilli

½ teaspoon saffron strands or ¼ teaspoon powder

Pinch salt substitute

½oz/15g butter

1 tablespoon hot water

2 tablespoons Greek strained yogurt or sour cream

Pinch cayenne, celery
  leaves or watercress
  to garnish

Place each chicken portion on a large piece of foil.
Melt saffron in the water and brush over chicken
thoroughly. Mix together garlic, spices, salt substitute and butter and divide between the two
portions. Dribble any remaining saffron over and
fold foil into two loose, airtight parcels. Bake at
180°C (350°F/Gas Mark 4) for 30 minutes or until
breasts are tender and cooked through. Serve on
Orange Rice (see below) with a tablespoon of
yogurt dribbled over each serving and garnished
with a pinch cayenne and a few celery or watercress leaves.

Orange Rice (Day 1)
130 calories per portion

2 oz/50 g (raw weight)   2 fl oz/50 ml chicken
  brown rice   stock
3 fl oz/75 ml orange   ½ oz/15 g sultanas
  juice   ½″ piece cinnamon
Grated rind of ½   (whole)
  orange   Pinch salt substitute

Simmer all ingredients in a small, tightly-lidded
saucepan for 30 minutes (or length of time
instructed on packet — brown rice cooking times

vary greatly). Add a little extra water towards end of cooking time if rice is getting too dry.

Honeyed Chicken (Day 1)
250 calories per portion

2 medium breast of chicken portions, skin removed
1″ garlic purée
1 tablespoon runny honey
2 tablespoons red wine vinegar
1 level teaspoon ground coriander
1 tablespoon olive or corn oil
2 teaspoons soya sauce

Mix everything except the chicken together well and coat the chicken pieces thoroughly with the mixture. Leave to marinade for at least 30 minutes then cook them under a medium grill for approx. 30 minutes, basting frequently with the surplus marinade.

Italian Fish Steaks (Day 2)
210 calories per portion

2 × 6 oz/175 g cod (or other white fish) steaks or fillets
2 oz/50 g button mushrooms, sliced
1 teaspoon (5 ml) cornflour
1 dessertspoon olive oil
1 teaspoon (5 ml) brown sugar

1″ garlic purée
4 fl oz/100 ml fish stock
  from cube
Small (7.5 oz) can
  chopped Italian
  tomatoes

½ teaspoon oregano
Pinch each black
  pepper, salt
  substitute
Dash Tabasco
  (optional)

Combine all ingredients except fish and mushrooms in a small bowl. Place fish steaks side by side in a shallow ovenproof casserole. Arrange mushrooms on top and pour over the sauce. Bake at 180°C (350°F/Gas Mark 4) for 30 minutes, tightly covered.

Sole in Mushroom Sauce (Day 2)
180 calories per portion

2 × 6 oz/175 g lemon
  sole fillets
6 oz/175 g button
  mushrooms, sliced
7 fl oz/200 ml skimmed
  milk

1 level tablespoon
  cornflour
Salt substitute and
  black pepper
Dash lemon juice

Poach the fish fillets in a frying pan in most of the milk for approx. 5 minutes. Mix the remaining milk with the cornflour. When the fillets are cooked, remove to a serving dish. Add the cornflour mixture to the milk in the frying pan with seasoning to taste and bring to boil, stirring constantly.

Add mushrooms and lemon juice and cook for further 2-3 minutes. Taste for seasoning; pour sauce over fish and serve.

Moroccan Lamb (Day 3)
300 calories per portion

8 oz/225 g lean lamb fillet, cubed
1 small onion, very finely chopped
1 clove garlic, crushed, or 1″ garlic purée
3 oz/75 g dried apricots
4 oz/100 g aubergine, cubed
1 dessertspoon corn oil
5 fl oz/150 ml beef stock
1 dessertspoon (10 ml) tomato purée
1 teaspoon (5 g) cornflour
½ teaspoon cumin
½ teaspoon ground coriander
Black pepper and salt substitute
1 dessertspoon apricot jam
1 tablespoon natural yogurt

Heat oil in non-stick frying pan and stir-fry lamb cubes until golden. Transfer to medium casserole. Stir-fry onions and garlic until soft and transparent. Transfer to casserole. Add apricots, aubergine, spices and seasoning to taste. Mix beef stock with the tomato purée and cornflour and pour into casserole. Bake at 170°C (325°F/Gas Mark 3) for 1 hour or until lamb is very tender and you have a thick sauce. (If too dry you can add a little extra beef stock or water towards end of cooking time, but there is not supposed to be much sauce.) Before serving, stir in the yogurt and jam.

Braised Citrus Beef (Day 3)
275 calories per portion

2 × 6 oz/175 g pieces extra lean braising steak
1 medium onion, puréed in a blender or very finely chopped
Good bunch parsley, chopped

½" garlic purée
Grated rind and juice of 1 large orange
Pinch chilli
Little salt substitute and black pepper
Dash Worcestershire sauce

In a small casserole or gratin dish, mix together all the ingredients except the beef. Add the steaks and baste thoroughly, leaving to marinade for at least 2 hours; longer if possible. Cook, covered in a 180°C (350°F/Gas Mark 4) oven for approx. 1¼ hours or until steaks are tender.

Chicken, Rice and Beansprout Salad (Day 4)
300 calories per portion (serves 1)

3 oz/75 g cooked chicken, skinned and diced

½ oz/15 g dried peaches ('no need to soak'), chopped OR sultanas

3 oz/75 g boiled brown
  rice
3 oz/75 g fresh
  beansprouts
2 oz/50 g green
  pepper, chopped
1 stick celery,
  chopped

2 fl oz/50 ml low-fat
  natural yogurt
1 teaspoon lemon juice
Black pepper and salt
  substitute
Good pinch turmeric or
  mild curry powder

Combine yogurt, lemon juice, seasoning to taste
and turmeric. Mix rest of ingredients into the
dressing. Turn onto serving plate, garnished with
salad leaves if liked.

Fennel Trout (Day 4)
255 calories per portion

2 × 7-8 oz/200-225 g
  prepared whole
  trout
Good bunch fennel
  leaves OR 2
  teaspoons fennel
  seeds

1 dessertspoon corn
  oil
1 fl oz (25 ml) dry white
  wine
1/2 a lemon
Pinch garam masala
Salt substitute and
  black pepper

Season the trout inside and out with the salt
substitute, pepper and garam masala. Put some
fennel leaves (or the seeds) inside each trout and
place each fish on a square of foil large enough to

make a parcel, first brushing the inside of the foil with the corn oil to prevent sticking. Divide the wine between the fish, add a dash of lemon juice to each then fold the foil up round each fish to make two loose, but airtight parcels. Bake at 220°C (440°F/Gas Mark 7) for 15 minutes or until trout are cooked through. Serve the fish in the foil, each with a lemon wedge.

Chicken Paprika (Day 5)
315 calories per portion

2 medium chicken portions, skinned
1 small onion, finely chopped
1 green pepper, de-seeded and sliced
3 fl oz/75 ml Greek strained yogurt
1 tablespoon corn oil

1 small (7.5 oz) tin chopped tomatoes
3 fl oz/75 ml chicken stock
1 teaspoon cornflour
1 heaped dessertspoon sweet paprika
Black pepper
Salt substitute to taste

Heat oil in a non-stick frying pan and stir-fry onion until soft and transparent. Place chicken portions in small casserole with the onion and arrange peppers on top. Mix together the tomatoes, stock, cornflour and paprika and add to casserole. Season to taste. Bake, covered, at 180°C (350°F/Gas Mark 4) for 45 minutes or until chicken is tender. Stir in the yogurt before serving.

Sherried Turkey (Day 5)
300 calories per portion

2 × 5oz/150g turkey
   fillets OR
   veal escallopes
1 level tablespoon olive
   oil
1 medium red pepper,
   de-seeded and sliced
   into very thin rings

1 small (7oz/200g) tin
   chopped tomatoes
1 glass medium dry
   sherry
1 tablespoon parsley,
   chopped
Salt substitute and
   black pepper

In a non-stick frying pan, heat the oil and fry the turkey fillets over a fairly high heat for a minute to brown each side. Remove from pan, lower heat and add pepper slices to pan. Fry for a few minutes until softened. Add sherry to pan, increase heat and allow to bubble, then add rest of ingredients including turkey, cover and simmer for 10 minutes or until fillets are cooked through. Check seasoning and serve the fillets with the sauce poured over.

Stir-Fried Beef in Oyster Sauce (Day 6)
310 calories per portion

8oz/225g extra-lean
   rump steak, sliced
   into thin bite-sized
   strips

½" garlic purée
   (optional)
1 dessertspoon dry or
   medium sherry

4 oz/100 g carrots, cut into matchsticks
4 oz/100 g whole beans, topped, tailed and cut into 2″ pieces
4 oz/100 g sweetcorn

1 teaspoon cornflour
1 dessertspoon corn oil
1 tablespoon oyster sauce
Little beef stock
1 teaspoon soya sauce

Combine the oyster sauce, garlic purée, cornflour, sherry, soya sauce and 2 tablespoons beef stock in a dish. Heat oil in wok or non-stick frying pan and when really hot, add meat, carrots and beans, stirring constantly. Stir 2 minutes. Add sweetcorn and stock mixture and continue stirring for 2-3 minutes. If mixture sticks or looks very dry, add more beef stock or water. Serve immediately. If you are watching calories, this would go well on a bed of lightly-boiled beansprouts. If not, serve with boiled brown rice or noodles.

NOTE: Oyster sauce is widely available at delis, supermarkets and speciality shops. It has a rich meaty flavour but doesn't taste of oysters!

Mushroom Pilau (Day 6)
340 calories per portion

5 oz/150 g (raw weight) brown rice
8 oz/225 g mushrooms, sliced

1 bay leaf
½ teaspoon cinnamon
1 tablespoon chopped parsley

1 egg, hard-boiled and quartered

1 oz/25 g sultanas or chopped dates

½ pint (10 fl oz/250 ml) vegetable stock

½" garlic purée

½" piece fresh ginger

1 level teaspoon each ground coriander, turmeric, cumin and paprika

2 tablespoons natural low-fat yogurt

1" piece cucumber, chopped

Little salt substitute and black pepper

1 dessertspoon oyster sauce

Few drops corn oil

In a lidded non-stick pan, heat the oil and add all the spices. Stir and cook over medium heat for a minute. Add the mushrooms and sultanas, stir. Add the rice, stir, then add most of the stock, the oyster sauce and a little salt substitute. Bring to simmer, stir, cover and simmer for approx. 18 minutes or until rice is cooked. Check after 10 minutes and add little more stock if rice looks too dry. Before serving, check seasoning then garnish the pilau with the egg pieces and the parsley.

Liver Stir-Fry (Day 7)
275 calories per portion

6 oz/175 g lamb's liver, cut into thin strips

8 oz/225 g broccoli florets

2 teaspoons cornflour

1 teaspoon brown sugar

2 fl oz/50 ml beef stock

4 oz/100 g leek,
   shredded
2 teaspoons corn oil
2 tablespoons red wine

Black pepper and salt
   substitute to taste
Chopped chives

Combine beef stock, cornflour, and sugar in cup.
Heat oil in wok or non-stick frying pan until really
hot. Add broccoli florets and stir-fry for 2-3
minutes. Add leeks and liver and stir-fry for one
minute. Add wine and let it bubble. Add stock
mixture, stir-fry for further minute. Season to taste
and add a little more stock if necessary. The stir-fry
shouldn't be too dry. Serve garnished with chopped
chives.

Nutty Red Peppers (Day 7)
330 calories per portion

1 large or 2 small red
   peppers
10 oz/25 g wholemeal
   breadcrumbs
2 oz/50 g chopped
   almonds
2 oz/50 g Mozzarella
   cheese, chopped
1 small (7 oz/200 g) can
   chopped tomatoes

4 oz/100 g mushrooms,
   chopped
1 fl oz/25 ml red wine
1/2 teaspoon chopped
   fresh basil or pinch
   dried basil
Little vegetable stock
Salt substitute and
   black pepper

Halve the pepper(s) lengthways and de-seed it,

then blanch in boiling water for 2 minutes and put halves in a suitable ovenproof dish. In a mixing bowl, combine all the rest of the ingredients, keeping back half the cheese and breadcrumbs. The mixture should be moist but not over-wet. Stuff the peppers with this mixture then top with the remaining cheese and breadcrumbs, mixed. Bake, without lid, at 190°C (375°F/Gas Mark 5) for approx. 45 minutes or until peppers are tender and topping is golden and sizzling.

Monkfish Kebabs (Day 8)
320 calories per portion

12 oz/325 g monkfish (or cod) fillet, cubed
8 oz/225 g green pepper, deseeded and cut into squares
3 tomatoes, cut into quarters
1 tablespoon olive oil
1 tablespoon red wine vinegar
1 tablespoon tomato purée
1 teaspoon Worcestershire sauce
1 dessertspoon clear honey
1″ garlic purée
1 level dessertspoon French mustard
1 teaspoon cornflour
1 fl oz/25 ml water
1 teaspoon basil
Black pepper

Combine everything except the fish and vegetables in a small saucepan and simmer gently while kebabs cook. Thread fish, peppers and tomatoes onto kebab sticks and brush with a little of the sauce. Grill kebabs under a medium/high heat for 12 minutes, turning once or twice. Serve with the sauce poured over.

Tangy Plaice (Day 8)
265 calories per portion

2 × 8oz/225g plaice fillets
1 small orange
1 small lemon

Half a glass (2½fl oz/ 60ml) dry white wine
1 teaspoon soya sauce
¼oz/10g butter
1 bay leaf

Cut two slices off the orange and the lemon then squeeze the juice from the remaining portions and mix with the wine, soya sauce and bay leaf. Put the plaice fillets in a large shallow dish and pour over the citrus mixture. Leave to marinade for half an hour. Cook the fillets on a medium to high grill, first brushing them with the melted butter. (Brush the rack with oil or butter too to prevent the fillets sticking.) Meanwhile, bring the remaining marinade to a boil in a small pan and reduce to half original quantity. When fillets are cooked (approx. 6 minutes) serve topped with the sauce and garnished with a slice of lemon and orange each.

Chicken Satay with Peanut Sauce (Day 9)
385 calories per portion

2 medium chicken
   breast fillets, skinned
   and cubed
Marinade:
1 tablespoon corn oil
1 tablespoon soya
   sauce
1 tablespoon tomato
   purée
1" garlic purée

For the sauce:
1 dessertspoon corn oil
1/2" garlic purée
1/2 teaspoon ground
   ginger
3 fl oz/75 ml water
1 1/2 tablespoons
   peanut butter
1 teaspoon tomato
   ketchup
1 teaspoon lemon juice
Dash Tabasco
Black pepper

Mix together the marinade ingredients in a bowl.
Add chicken, mix and leave as long as possible —
preferably overnight, but 3 hours will do. Then
thread chicken onto four wooden skewers and grill
under a medium heat for 15 minutes, turning once
or twice. Meanwhile, make the sauce. Combine all
the ingredients in a small saucepan and simmer
gently, stirring from time to time. Serve in a small
side dish with the satay sticks, garnished with
salad leaves or spring onions if liked.

Stuffed Chicken Breasts (Day 9)
335 calories per portion

2 medium chicken
  breast portions,
  skin left on, boned
1 small onion, puréed
  in blender
1 oz/25 g shelled
  walnuts, chopped
3 oz/75 g mushrooms,
  chopped

1 dessertspoon olive oil
Little chicken stock
Dash mushroom
  ketchup
Dash lemon juice
Little salt substitute
  and black pepper
1 tablespoon parsley,
  chopped

In a small non-stick frying pan, cook the onion in the oil for a few minutes, then add the mushrooms, cook for a further few minutes, then add the rest of the stuffing ingredients and cook gently for five more minutes, stirring from time to time. Meanwhile gently lift the chicken skins from the flesh, leaving one side attached. When the stuffing mixture has cooled a little, pack it in under the skin and secure either with wooden toothpicks or by sewing. Now grill the breasts over a pan to catch the juices for approx. 30 minutes under a medium heat or until breasts are nicely browned and cooked right through. Serve with any juices in pan.

Stuffed Aubergine (Day 10)
500 calories per portion

1 very large or 2 small
  aubergines

1 dessertspoon tomato
  purée

8 oz/225 g extra-lean minced beef

1 medium onion, very finely chopped

1 clove garlic, chopped, OR 1″ garlic purée

Good pinch nutmeg

1 dessertspoon corn oil

4 fl oz/100 ml beef stock

2 oz/50 g Edam cheese, grated

Black pepper

½ teaspoon salt substitute

Green salad leaves

Cut aubergine(s) in half lengthways and scoop out pulp. Sprinkle both skins and flesh with salt and leave to drain in colander for an hour. Wash and rinse off salt and pat dry. (This takes away any slight bitterness the aubergine may have.) Heat oil in non-stick pan and stir-fry onion and garlic until soft and just turning gold. Add beef and brown. Drain off any fat that you can. Add nutmeg, tomato purée mixed with the stock, pepper and salt substitute and simmer for 10 minutes. Combine the beef mixture with the aubergine flesh, chopped. Place the aubergine skins in an ovenproof dish and fill with the beef mixture. Put a very little water in the bottom of the dish, cover and bake at 180°C (350°F/Gas Mark 4) for 30 minutes or until aubergines are tender. Sprinkle cheese over top and brown under grill. Serve with a green salad.

Minty Lamb Kebabs (Day 10)
320 calories per portion

10 oz/275 g extra lean fillet of lamb, cubed
1 level dessertspoon mild curry paste
½ teaspoon ground ginger
Juice of ½ a lemon
5 or 6 sprigs fresh mint, chopped
Good teaspoon runny honey
Dash Tabasco
½" garlic purée
1 tablespoon red wine vinegar
Little salt substitute
5 fl oz/150 ml natural low-fat yogurt

In a bowl, combine the curry paste, ginger and lemon juice and add the lamb, mixing all well. Leave to marinade for as long as possible, but at least an hour or two. Thread the lamb onto kebab sticks and grill, turning occasionally, for approx. 15 minutes. Meanwhile, beat all the remaining ingredients together well in a small bowl, check for seasoning and serve at room temperature with the kebabs.

Lentil Soup (Day 11)
250 calories per portion

4 oz/100 g brown lentils
1 pint vegetable stock
2 oz/50 g potato, cut into small cubes
2 oz/50 g carrot, sliced
1 small onion, finely chopped
Black pepper
Salt substitute to taste

Put all ingredients in saucepan and simmer, covered, for 1½ hours or until lentils are tender (times will vary considerably — may be much less than this, or a little longer, depending upon how old the lentils are). Put the soup through an electric blender for a thick soup, adding a little more stock or water if necessary, or serve as a chunky soup if preferred.

Veal and Aubergine Casserole (Day 11)
240 calories per portion

10 oz/300 g fillet of veal (or pork), cubed

1 average (10 oz/300 g) aubergine

1 small onion, finely chopped

1 small (7 oz/200 g) tin tomatoes

1 level tablespoon tomato purée

1 teaspoon ground cumin

Few sage leaves

4 fl oz/100 ml chicken stock

Salt substitute and black pepper

¼ oz/10 g butter

Slice the aubergine, sprinkle with salt and leave to drain in a colander for at least 30 minutes. Rinse well and dry with kitchen paper. Melt the butter in a non-stick frying pan and gently cook the onion until it is soft. Remove, add veal, turn up heat and brown for a minute, stirring. Transfer all ingredients to a casserole dish and cook, covered, so that it barely simmers, for approx. 1 hour at 150°G (300°F/Gas Mark 2).

Baked Egg Ratatouille (Day 12)
275 calories per portion

2 eggs size 3
8 oz/225 g aubergine including skin, chopped
4 oz/100 g green pepper, deseeded and sliced
8 oz/225 g courgettes, sliced
1/4 oz/10 g butter

1 small onion, finely chopped
1 small (7.5 oz) tin tomatoes
2 tablespoons olive oil
2 teaspoons ground coriander
Black pepper
Salt substitute to taste

Heat the oil in a non-stick frying pan and stir-fry all the vegetables except the tomatoes, for 5 minutes. Add seasoning, cover and simmer very slowly for 30 minutes, stirring from time to time. Add tomatoes and cook for further 20-30 minutes until all vegetables are tender. Divide the ratatouille between two individual shallow ovenproof dishes. Make a well in the centre of each mixture and break an egg into each. Sprinkle on a little black pepper, dot each egg with a tiny knob of butter, and bake at 180°C (350°F/Gas Mark 4) until eggs are set — about 15 minutes.

Courgette Gratin (Day 12)
270 calories per portion

10 oz/275 g courgettes
2 oz/50 g rye or
  wholemeal
  breadcrumbs
2 oz/50 g Gruyère
  cheese, grated

Small (7 oz/200 g)
  tin tomatoes
1 level tablespoon
  olive oil
1 teaspoon basil
Black pepper

Slice the courgettes into ¼″ rounds and sauté them in the oil in a non-stick pan until golden brown. Now add the tomatoes and seasoning, cover and simmer for 15 minutes. Transfer to individual gratin dishes, top with the cheese and breadcrumbs mixed together and put under a medium grill for approx. 10 minutes until topping is golden.

Salad Soup (Day 13)
50 calories per portion

1 large (15 oz) can
  tomatoes, chopped
8 oz/225 g cucumber,
  chopped small
1 × 6 oz/175 g green
  pepper, deseeded
  and chopped
1 clove garlic, crushed

1 tablespoon red wine
  vinegar
Dash Tabasco
Black pepper
Salt substitute to taste
Ice cubes
Tomato juice as
  necessary

Keep back a few pieces of cucumber and pepper. Blend the remaining ingredients (except extra tomato juice) in an electric blender — if you would prefer a thinner soup, add a little tomato juice and reblend. Chill for 3 hours, check seasoning, serve garnished with chopped pepper and cucumber and ice cubes.

Salmon in Lemon Cream (Day 13)
370 calories per portion

2 × 4oz/100g salmon steaks	Half a lemon
4floz/100ml single cream	2 sprigs parsley
½oz/15g butter	Little salt substitute and black pepper

Put the steaks in a small buttered ovenproof dish so that they fit tightly. Season with salt substitute and pepper. Peel the lemon and slice, and place the slices over the salmon. Now pour over the cream and bake at 190°C (375°F/Gas Mark 5) for approx. 15-20 minutes, if necessary, basting the tops of the salmon with cream to stop them from drying. Serve with the cream sauce, garnished with parsley.

Ginger Chicken (Day 14)
365 calories per portion

8 oz/225 g lean chicken meat, cut into strips

2 oz/50 g sweetcorn

6 oz/175 g mushrooms, sliced

¼ oz/10 g piece fresh ginger, peeled

2 oz/50 g (dry weight) noodles

4 oz/100 g mangetout

1 tablespoon dry or medium sherry

1 dessertspoon soya sauce

2 fl oz/50 ml chicken stock

1 teaspoon cornflour

Salt substitute to taste

Heat oil in wok or non-stick frying pan. Add mangetout and stir-fry for 2 minutes. Add chicken, sweetcorn, mushrooms and ginger, stir-fry for another 2 minutes. Add sherry; allow to bubble. Add stock mixed with cornflour and soya sauce; stir until sauce thickens. Meanwhile put noodles in a pan of boiling water and allow to stand for 2 minutes. Just before serving, gently mix the boiled noodles with the chicken and vegetables. Remove the piece of ginger before serving.

NOTE: for a stronger ginger flavour, chop the ginger finely and leave it in the finished dish.

Liver with Sage (Day 14)
290 calories per portion

8 oz/225 g calves'
　or lamb's liver,
　thinly sliced
1 small onion, puréed
　in blender
1 tablespoon corn oil

1 tablespoon chopped
　fresh sage
2 fl oz/50 ml chicken
　stock
2 fl oz/50 ml red wine
Salt substitute and
　black pepper

Put the onion, stock, wine, a little seasoning and half
the sage into a saucepan, bring to boil and cook for
10-15 minutes until it has reduced to a gravy-like
consistency. Meanwhile, heat a grill or a non-stick
pan. Brush the liver with the oil, sprinkle on the remaining sage, and grill or fry on high for 2-3 minutes
a side; no more. Serve liver with sauce poured over.

Mustard Steak (Day 15)
400 calories per portion

2 × 5 oz/150 g fillet or
　rump steaks, extra
　lean
½ oz/15 g butter
Black pepper

4 fl oz/100 ml Greek
　strained yogurt
2 good teaspoons
　French mustard
　(preferably Dijon)

Heat the butter in a non-stick frying pan, and when
sizzling but not brown, add the steaks and cook on
high for 3-5 minutes a side, depending upon the
thickness and your own preference. When cooked,

remove steaks on a slatted spatula to serving plate and keep warm. Add the yoghurt, mustard and pepper to the pan and stir to warm through but don't let the yoghurt boil. Serve immediately under the steaks.

Lentil Bolognese with Pasta (Day 15)
480 calories per portion

4 oz/100 g green or brown lentils
1 medium onion, puréed in blender
½" garlic purée
2 sticks celery, finely chopped
1 carrot, finely chopped
1 small (7 oz/200 g) can chopped tomatoes
1 tablespoon olive oil
1 tablespoon tomato purée
1 teaspoon marjoram
5 fl oz/150 ml vegetable stock
4 oz/100 g dry weight wholewheat pasta
2 level dessertspoons grated Parmesan cheese

Boil the lentils in plenty of water until tender — about an hour, or less depending upon their age. Drain. In a non-stick frying pan, sauté the celery, onion and carrot in the oil for a few minutes, stirring. Add the garlic, tomatoes, tomato purée, marjoram and stock, bring to boil and simmer for 30 minutes until sauce is a good, thick consistency. Check for taste, adding a little salt substitute if necessary. Meanwhile boil the pasta in plenty of water and serve with the Lentil Bolognese and Parmesan cheese.

CHAPTER FIVE

The Flat Stomach Exercises

Without strong 'abdominals', your stomach will never be really flat. And, unlike the other major muscle groups of your body, your stomach muscles don't get much work in day-to-day, normal activity, so you have to make a conscious effort to keep them in condition.

I used to think that this was a hopeless task, but I now know that many of the exercises I used to do were virtually useless. In fact, many of the exercises still around and promoted as the best ones for the stomach are not *only* almost useless — they can be dangerous, too.

Useless because they don't position you correctly and so they exercise other parts of your body more than your stomach — the tops of your thighs, for instance. And *dangerous* because of the strain they place on your back when your back is probably too weak to cope. The classic straight-leg sit up is a perfect example of a 'stomach' exercise that's both over-rated for the purpose — and tough on your back. Also it does nothing whatsoever for the 'oblique' muscles that criss-cross your midriff and give your waist its definition.

The exercises in my programme give a complete and *safe* workout to the *whole* stomach area from chest to hips and side to side — even your back view will improve, too!

As you do the exercise plan, you will notice improvement starting *first* under the bust and around the waist. The improvement works *downwards*. So don't, after a few days, say 'it isn't working' — just continue with the programme and it *will* work.

USING THE PROGRAMME

The grade system

My Flat Stomach Workout looks simple — because it *is* simple. I'm not saying you will find the routine takes no effort — if it were that easy, it wouldn't work. But because of the special system I've devised, it will suit your level of capability perfectly. It will be no more and no less than *you* need.

Whether your stomach muscles — and your general fitness — are poor, very poor — or absolutely terrible! — you can use the programme with confidence with its unique grade system for each stomach exercise.

You start the programme on Grade 1, which is the easiest. You progress from Grade 1 through to Grade 3 during the fifteen-day programme. Grade 2 is hard, Grade 3 is hardest — but as you are progressing in a sensible way, by the time you start Grade 2, and then Grade 3, they won't *seem* too hard.

All I ask is that you give your very best to the programme, and it will do the rest for you.

All you do is begin on Grade 1 for each exercise — and, when you can do that grade without difficulty, move on to Grade 2, and then to Grade 3. As soon as you can do a grade — don't linger, move up! That's the way to a flat stomach. But DON'T move up too quickly, before you are ready.

If you have very weak stomach muscles, you may stay on Grade 1 for a week, for at least some of the exercises. If you aren't so weak, you may move to Grade 2 after three or four days, and be able to do Grade 3 by the end of the first week.

Think positive and you'll be surprised by what you CAN do. To progress you must stretch yourself — but listen to your body and don't push *too* hard.

The routine

The programme consists of a WARM-UP, SIX STOMACH EXERCISES, each preceded by a pelvic tilt and followed by a knees-in, four COUNTER-BALANCING exercises and finally a COOL DOWN.

The whole workout should take you no more than forty minutes a day, and never less than thirty.

To anyone who is now saying 'That seems a lot of time to find,' I can only say, think of all the time you have wasted on other programmes; think of all the time you have wasted worrying about the way your body looks. *All I ask is forty minutes a day for fifteen days for you to see fantastic results*.

Because it is essential for you to know WHY you are doing these particular exercises, and even more essential to know HOW to do them properly — it is *vital* that you *read all the notes that follow* both here, and accompanying each exercise photo. If you do the routine without paying enough attention to the notes, *you won't achieve the results both you and I want*.

First let's talk you through the routine.

The warm-up

This is essential — your body isn't ready for work until it is warmed up. Warming up means your circulation improves, your major muscles get warm and more supple. Without a warm-up even simple exercises can seem much harder and you run the risk of straining yourself. So *do* the warm-up — it doesn't take long and it will make the whole programme much more pleasant and safe.

The stomach exercises 1-6

These are for the different muscle groups that define your upper and lower abdomen and your waist. Start on Grade 1 for each of these exercises. As soon as you can do the number of repeats and/or the length of 'hold' given for each exercise without difficulty, move up a grade. When you can do the Grade 3 exercises without difficulty you can, if you wish, increase the number of repeats/length of 'hold' given.

Make sure to read the instructions for these exercises carefully before you begin. They are vital. Preceding each stomach exercise you do a pelvic tilt — a simple movement that takes seconds, but is essential because it aligns you correctly. After each of the stomach exercises you do a knees-in — a movement which will help prevent strain and will help you do the programme easily.

The counter-balancing exercises 7-10

These achieve two purposes: one, to stretch and relax the stomach muscles that have been doing all the hard work and two, to help strengthen and mobilise your lower back and hips. In people with weak stomach muscles, these are often problem areas which need to be worked on alongside the stomach exercises for really good results. They will also help your posture — for more on which, see Chapter 6.

After the intensive stomach work, you will find these exercises pleasant to do. Don't skip them. They each have only one grade which you stay on throughout the fifteen days.

The cool-down

This is a wonderful way to end the session — a five-minute long body stretch that, I can assure you, feels marvellous. Apart from cooling you down and relaxing you, it is also a fabulous exercise in itself, especially for people with posture problems and/or who spend long hours hunched over desks. It stretches out tensions in neck and shoulders, improves the bustline and breathing, stretches out the ribcage and midriff, lengthens the waist and flattens the stomach — all while you 'just lie there' and let gravity help you! In fact, it is vital you do the long body stretch properly so do read the instructions for that exercise carefully.

At the end of your workout you should feel GOOD. You should also feel as though you have made an effort — nicely tired and stretched in every sense of the word. If you feel as if you have done nothing, you're not putting enough into the programme. Try harder tomorrow.

Before you begin

Here are my guidelines to help you get the most from your programme. Don't skip these, either!

The room

Choose a quiet room with enough space to carry out the exercises properly — this means a space at least 8 ft by 6 ft. The floor should be carpeted or else you will need to use an exercise mat. Cover the carpet or mat with a thick towel for added comfort and hygiene. You may find a small, flat cushion useful for supporting your head during exercises 1-6. This won't detract from their effectiveness.

You will need a sturdy dining chair or large stool of chair height. It will also help to have a full-length mirror to check posture and improvement but this isn't essential. The room should be warm — around 70°C. If you exercise in a cold room you risk muscle strain — warm muscles perform much more easily. The exercise programme is not aerobic, so you won't get over-hot. You can have some background music if you like, but don't try to perform the exercises in time with music; they aren't designed that way.

Your clothes

Don't wear anything that restricts your movement. *Do* wear something so that you can see your body and what it is doing. A stretchy leotard is ideal; or a vest and lycra cycling shorts, or ordinary shorts and a T-shirt. You could wear a tracksuit to do the warm-up. Shoes are not essential for this routine, as you won't be doing any exercises that jar the feet or legs. In fact, I suggest you *don't* wear thick-soled trainers as the added height may throw some of the exercises out of balance. Pin long hair back or it might distract you.

The time

Ideally, do the programme at a set time every day. I find this helps because it is important not to miss a day and if you don't have a set time, twenty-four hours go so quickly it's easy to skip. It will help your body to be warmed up if you do the programme when you've been up a while, so don't leap straight out of bed and do it. Also, leave at least ninety minutes after a meal before beginning.

Familiarisation

You should spend one session of *more* than forty minutes getting to know the routine and making sure you understand what the movements are and how you do them. If you have a partner around to look at what you're doing, it is even better. The routine is simple so after a day or two you will not need to refer to the book all the time. But you *must* do the exercises right!

The movements

Forget all about fast, jerky movements. All the exercises in the Flat Stomach Programme are meant to be carried out in a slow, controlled and smooth way. They depend upon HOLDING positions as much as REPEATING movements. Keep thinking CONTROL. Throughout each of the exercises, and the warm-up and cool-down, you should be aware of your stomach and what it is doing. If you are asking too much of it, or aren't maintaining the pelvic tilt, it may bulge out — you'll be able to see easily if this is happening. Ease down a bit.

Breathe normally throughout unless instructed otherwise. Don't hold your breath. You will find it comes naturally to breathe in before a movement and out during the movement, but any breathing that doesn't seem natural should be avoided.

Safety

All the exercises are safe if you follow the instructions both here and with the exercise photos. I have paid particular attention to avoiding the exercises most likely to hurt your back.

Difficulties

Anyone of any ability in normal health should be able to master the programme without undue difficulty and without risk. As with any exercise programme, though, if you are receiving medical attention or have a particular physical problem or have not exercised for years, I advise you to consult your doctor before beginning the routine.

If you are very stiff, weak and/or out of condition you may find some of the exercises hard to carry out as shown at first. In this case, just do your best and with every day you will get better and they will get easier.

You shouldn't feel *pain* on doing the exercises — but you should feel you are working. On Day 2 you may feel some stiffness; persist with the programme and by Day 4 this will have gone, to be replaced by an increasing feeling of control and pleasure in your own body and strength.

On finishing

At the end of the fifteen days, turn to page 204 for what to do next.

Finally, remember your promise to me. You will do your best. Carry out the Flat Stomach Programme as a ballet dancer would do her exercises — with determination, dedication and concentration. Don't shirk! The programme will work — *if* you give it your all.

The pelvic tilt

You need to learn how to do this simple movement before you begin the routine as you will need to adopt the tilt before virtually every exercise, and attempt to maintain it throughout. It helps you do the exercises properly, and every time you do it, it improves your posture. Eventually it becomes second nature. And it's so easy.

Learn it lying down, but you can do it standing or sitting, too. It just means that your pelvis is aligned properly, not tipped forward, as is so often the case with most of us.

1. Lie down as shown (Figure 1). Put your hand under the small of your back; you will find a

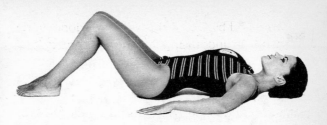

FIGURE 1

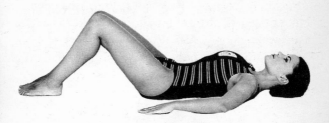

FIGURE 2

gap — maybe a big gap. The pelvic tilt will close this gap. Remove your hand and put arms by sides.

2. Make sure your neck and shoulders are flat on the ground — now, using your stomach muscles, press your low back down into the floor, and tilt your pubic bone towards your upper body. Your pelvis is now properly aligned (Figure 2). Pull your stomach *hard* towards the floor and hold it in for a count of five before beginning your exercise.

The knees-in

After exercises 1-6 you do a knees-in. This helps keep your body balanced throughout the routine.

1. Lie as shown, holding a pelvic tilt.
2. Now raise right leg and pull in with your hands clasped around knee; as far into your chest as knee will go, raising head slightly at the same time (Figure 3). Hold pull for count of ten. Repeat with the left leg. If your hip/groin area is especially inflexible, your knees will come closer and closer to your chest day by day as the programme helps you supple up.

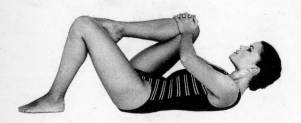

FIGURE 3

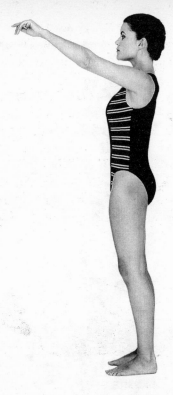

FIGURE 4

WARM-UP

1. Stand as shown and do 20 large arm circles from front to back with each arm in turn. Don't let head pull back; don't twist at hips; keep neck straight (Figures 4, 5, and 6).

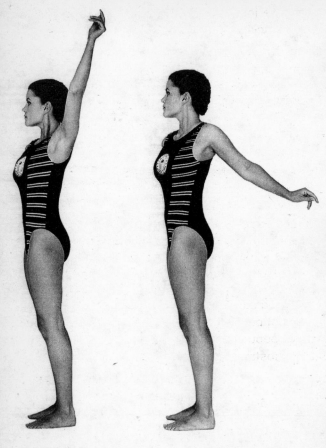

FIGURE 5

FIGURE 6

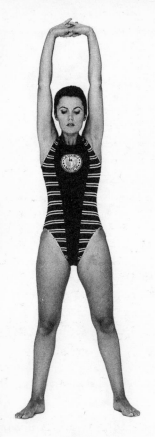

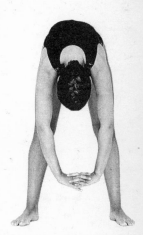

FIGURE 7   **FIGURE 8**

2. Stand as shown and clasp hands together over head (Figure 7). Swing down towards floor, keeping feet apart and knees bent (Figure 8). Continue

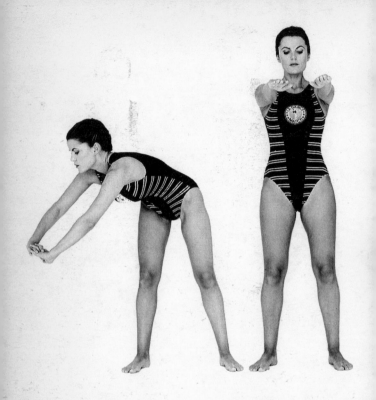

FIGURE 9   **FIGURE 10**

swing round to right (Figure 9) and made a big, rhythmic circle with your upper body until you are back at the floor position. Do 10 big circles to the right; then 10 to the left. If you're doing it right you should be breathing deeper at the end.

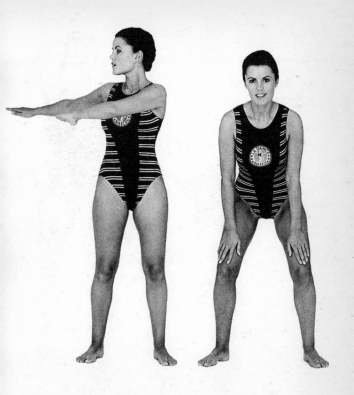

FIGURE 11   **FIGURE 12**

3. Stand as shown (Figure 10) and swing your body slowly to the right, keeping hips as still as possible (Figure 11). Now swing round to the left, looking in the direction you are swinging. Repeat the right/left movement 10 times.

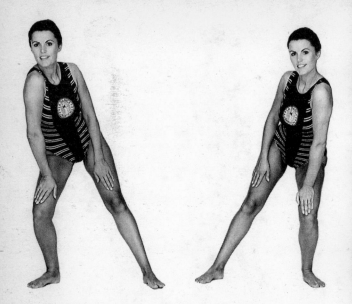

FIGURE 13   **FIGURE 14**

4. Stand as shown (Figure 12). Now in a rhythmic movement, bring first your right knee, hip and shoulder forward (Figure 13), then your left (Figure 14), keeping feet firmly in place. Repeat right/left movement 10 times.

5. Now stand as shown and swing out in front of you first your right leg then your left (Figure 15), in big, marching movements. Do 10 marches on each leg.

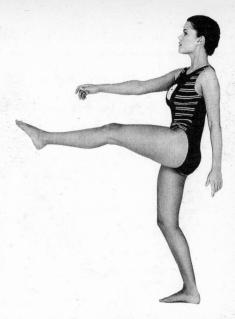

FIGURE 15

ONE: THE CURL UP

Grade 1

Lie on the floor as shown, knees slightly apart and feet firmly on the floor. Breathe steadily. Do a pelvic tilt (Figure 16). Now, making sure to hold the pelvic tilt position and concentrating on your stomach area throughout the exercise, slowly lift head, neck and arms off the floor (Figure 17). Hold the curl up for a count of 5, then slowly return to floor and repeat 10 times. Do a knees-in.

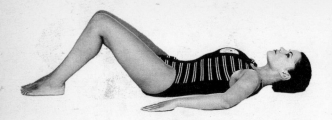

FIGURE 16

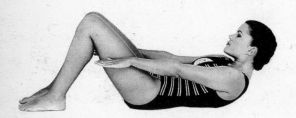

FIGURE 17

Important Curl head up before neck to prevent neck strain — don't let neck drag head up. A small cushion will help here. As you get stronger you may raise higher off floor up to 40° angle, but you will achieve nothing by curling up further — the stomach muscles of the upper and lower abdomen are used most in the first few inches of this movement. Don't use *any* pressure from arms, hands or legs to help lift you up. Your legs should remain relaxed and static throughout the exercise.

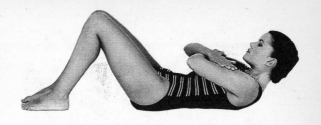

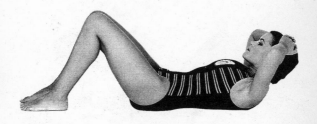

FIGURE 19

Grade 2
As Grade 1 but with arms folded across chest (Figure 18).

Grade 3
As Grade 1 but with hands placed over ears or on top of head (never on back of head) and with arms out wide (Figure 19).

TWO: THE CROSSED CURL

Grade 1

Lie as shown in curl-up position but arms out to sides (Figure 20). Do a pelvic tilt. Now slowly bring your right arm up and over your body towards your left hip, and bring it down to a point level with but as far to the left from your left hip as you can

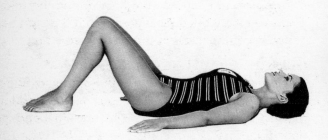

FIGURE 20

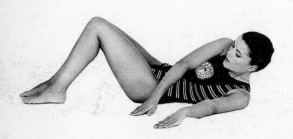

FIGURE 21

make it (Figure 21). Your right shoulder and upper body should come off the floor but your hips should remain on the floor. Hold the reach for a count of 2 then slowly relax back to floor and repeat 10 times. Repeat to right side then do a knees-in.

Important Do the movement slowly. Don't worry if you can't reach far at first — but give it your best. Every day you will do better. Don't use your 'free' arm to push into the floor during this exercise; all the work should come from the stomach and waist muscles on the side you're lifting.

Grade 2
This time lie on your left hip with right leg over left leg and right foot resting on floor as shown. Now move arms up and to the right and lift head off floor (Figure 22). Hold for count of 5. Return to floor. Repeat 10 times, turn over and repeat other side.

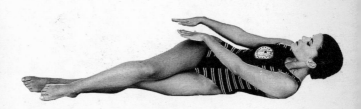

FIGURE 22

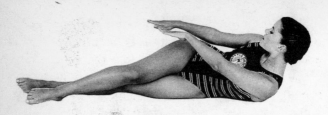

FIGURE 23

Grade 3
Same position as Grade 2, but this time curl up further until your shoulders are off the floor and hold for count of 5 (Figure 23). Repeat 10 times, repeat to other side.

THREE: CURL BACK

Grade 1
Sit up as shown, lower back straight and pelvis tilted correctly. Stretch arms out in front of you to either side of knees (Figure 24). Now, very very slowly curl backwards to maximum 45° (Figure 25). Hold for a count of 15. Move back to start and repeat 5 times. Lie down and do a knees-in.

> **Important** This is a marvellous exercise for your lower abdomen, but all the benefit is in doing the movement in a slow and controlled way. If you can't get all the way back to 45° and hold it for 15 at first, just go as far back as you can to hold.

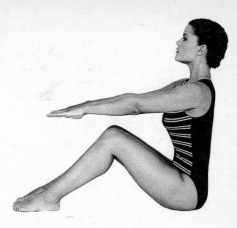

FIGURE 24

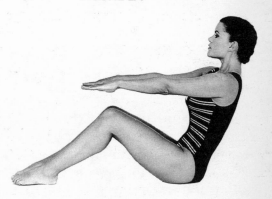

FIGURE 25

If you are slim you may find the base of your spine hurts as you roll back during this exercise. In that case use a double thickness of towel under you.

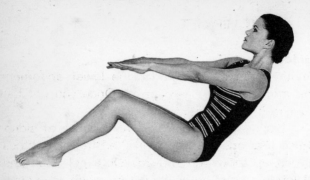

FIGURE 26

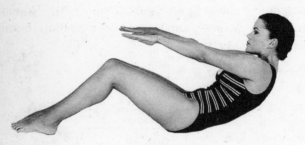

FIGURE 27

Grade 2

Curl on further back than at Grade 1 and hold for count of 25 (Figure 26). Slowly return to start — the return is equally important.

Grade 3

Curl all the way back to the floor — slowly, slowly (Figure 27). To get back to start for each repeat, use arms to push yourself up without jerking.

FOUR: HIP LIFT

Grade 1

Another marvellous one for the lower abdomen; the most stubborn area of all! Once you get the hang of it, it's not difficult at all.

Lie on the floor, knees bent, arms at sides. Raise first one leg and then the other and cross ankles, as shown (Figure 28). Do a pelvic tilt and maintain correct pelvic angle throughout. Now in a continuous, rhythmic movement, lift hips from floor and gently lower them back (Figure 29). Repeat 10 times; lower legs and do a knees-in, then repeat a further 10 times.

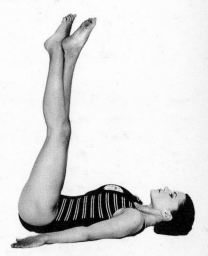

FIGURE 28

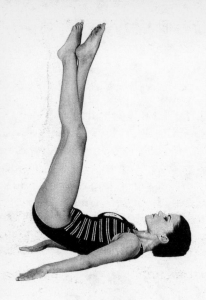

FIGURE 29

Important Don't try to lock knees on this one. Don't let legs creep back down towards floor while you do the exercise — if anything they should be pointing towards your head. Don't use arm pressure to help push your hips up; all the lift should come from your abdomen.

Grade 2
Cross your arms over your lower belly, making sure elbows don't touch floor (Figure 30). Carry out exercise as in Grade 1.

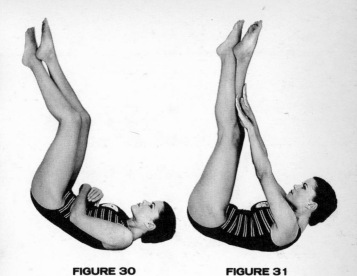

FIGURE 30 **FIGURE 31**

Grade 3

Reach your arms up to grab knees and lift head slightly off floor (Figure 31). Carry out exercise as in Grade 1.

FIVE: DIAGONAL LIFTS

Grade 1

Lie on back as shown with feet on wall and legs making a 90° angle, hands on ears, elbows out. Do a pelvic tilt (Figure 32).

Raise your right arm and shoulder up and across your body and as you do so, bring in your

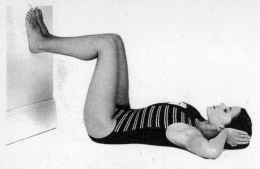

FIGURE 32

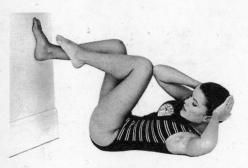

FIGURE 33

left knee to meet your elbow (Figure 33). Return to start and repeat other side. Do 10 of these 'cycling' movements each side. Do a knees-in.

   Important Keep elbows out for full benefit. Maintain correct pelvic tilt throughout.

Grade 2
Same starting position as Grade 1 this time, leave legs still with feet against wall and bring right side

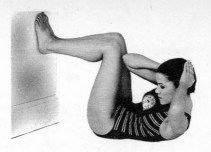

FIGURE 34

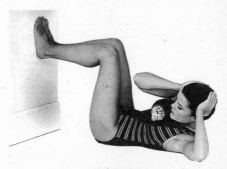

FIGURE 35

and elbow up until elbow touches left knee (Figure 34). Relax back and repeat to other side. Repeat 10 times.

Grade 3

Same starting position as Grade 1. Leave your legs where they are and bring your right side and arm up and over body and try to touch floor on left side with right elbow (Figure 35).

SIX: THE CRUNCH

Grade 1

Using a sturdy dining chair, sit as shown with ankles on edge of chair and hands supporting body on either side. Do a pelvic tilt. Attempt to rest as little weight on your hands as possible (Figure 36). Now, breathing out, move forward to touch your ankles, working your lower stomach muscles to keep yourself balanced (Figure 37). Hold for count of 2 then return to start. Repeat 10 times. Lie down and do a knees-in.

Important The chair should be the correct height. You should concentrate on keeping your

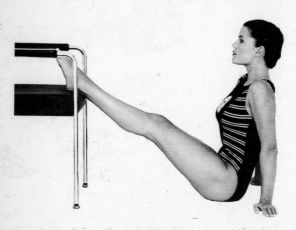

FIGURE 36

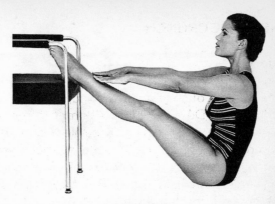

FIGURE 37

back up and balanced by using your stomach.
The more you do this exercise the less your
hands should be supporting you.

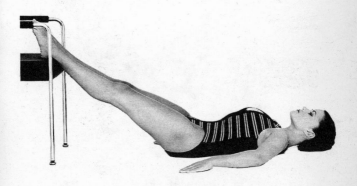

FIGURE 38

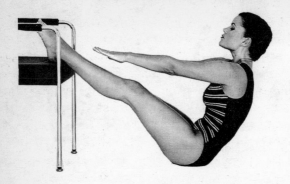

FIGURE 39

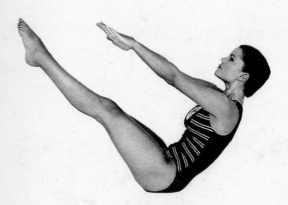

FIGURE 40

Grade 2

Lie on the floor, arms at sides, legs on chair as before (Figure 38). Now slowly lift yourself up to touch ankles as before (Figure 39).

Grade 3

This is a tough one. You may not reach this grade during the fifteen days, so be warned! Lie on floor in curl-up position, knees bent. Bring one leg then the other up into the air, straight, to 45°. Do the pelvic tilt then, on an out breath, stretch out arms towards legs and raise whole upper body in a flowing movement towards your ankles (Figure 40). Hold for count of 3; slowly lie back and repeat 5 times. Once you can do this, keep the hold for 10, then 15.

SEVEN: KNEELING LEG LIFT

Kneel on floor, arms and legs square as shown. Do a pelvic tilt to flatten back (Figure 41). Now, in a slow

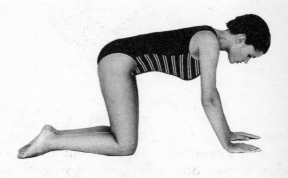

FIGURE 41

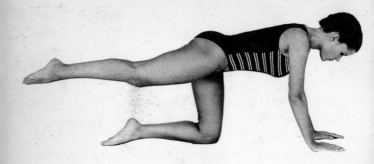

FIGURE 42

and controlled way, bring right leg up and out to the back until it is horizontal to the floor. Don't dip left hip; keep body level (Figure 42).

Clenching the buttock, hold the position for a count of 20. Return leg slowly to floor. Repeat other side. Arch back like a cat to finish.

EIGHT: COBRA AND CHILD

This movement is based on yoga positions; there are no repeats, you just hold positions and flow from one to the other. The sequence mobilises your back and stretches your front.

Lie on your front, upper body supported on elbows as shown. Hold the position for 30, keeping head and eyes up and breathing steadily (Figure 43).

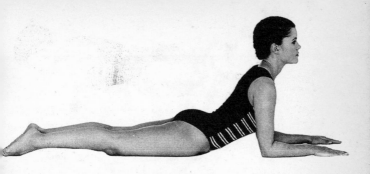

FIGURE 43

Relax to the floor and put arms under shoulders, palms flat on floor. Now push your upper body up until arms are straight, head up and only hands and legs touching floor. Hold for 30 (Figure 44).

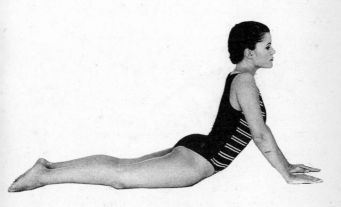

FIGURE 44

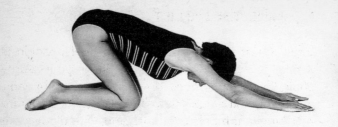

FIGURE 45

Now gradually slide your bottom backwards, keeping hands and knees on floor and bringing head down towards floor. When your arms and back make a straight 45° line, hold for 20 (Figure 45). Carry on back, sliding arms backwards slightly, until you are sitting on heels as shown (Figure 46). Hold for 20. Feel the stretch along your back through the latter part of this movement.

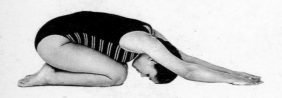

FIGURE 46

NINE: THE SKI LIFT

I call this the ski lift because the final position is similar to a racing ski position. Sit on your sturdy chair. Flop upper body down between your legs, arms loose at sides. Relax for 20 seconds (Figure 47). Now put hands over ears and, with elbows out to the sides, use your back to pull yourself slowly up to a 45° angle as shown (Figure 48). Hold for 20. Relax back down and repeat.

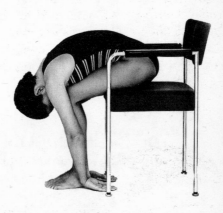

FIGURE 47

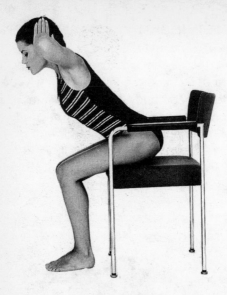

FIGURE 48

TEN: THE LUNGE

You will be lunging like a fencer in this one. Stand as shown, sliding right leg backwards as far as you can, and keeping left knee bent, left hand on knee. Slowly bounce a few inches up and down, trying to stretch the groin area as you go (Figure 49). Bounce gently 20 times. Repeat other side. You may hold onto the back of a chair by your side if you need a little balance support at first. If so, keep the chair on the side with your free hand and leg behind you.

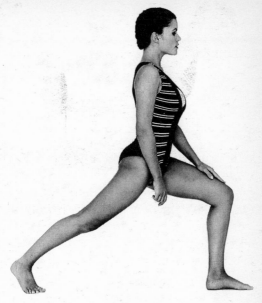

FIGURE 49

COOL DOWN

The long body stretch

Lie on your back, legs in the curl up position. Slowly raise your arms above your head until the backs of your palms touch the floor. The back of your neck should be as flat as possible; get someone to test how big the gap is between neck and

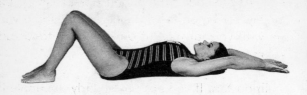

FIGURE 50

floor, if possible. Don't allow your chin to move upwards, towards your hands. You should maintain a pelvic tilt throughout. Now lie there for a minute, breathing a little more deeply than usual, and feel the stretch throughout your upper body — you should feel it in your shoulders, arms, ribcage and abdomen (Figure 50). Now wriggle each hip in turn to try to elongate your body even more, then slowly lower first one leg then the other so that you are lying flat. Lie there for a minimum of four minutes, relaxing yet stretching yourself out and keeping your stomach in (Figure 51).

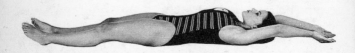

FIGURE 51

At the end of the period, don't rush up. Get up slowly, rolling on to your side and pushing yourself up with your arms. Put on a robe or tracksuit and relax for a few minutes.

Important If you are particularly unsupple in the neck, shoulders and back and/or round-shouldered, you will find it hard to keep your arms in the correct position without having your stomach — perhaps even your hips — come up off the floor. In this case, just try your best to get to the right position and day by day, gravity and your own increasing suppleness will help you get there.

CHAPTER SIX

Reinforcements

You're on the Flat Stomach Diet, and doing the exercise programme daily. This combination alone will work wonders on your shape.

But there is still more you can do to help that flat stomach along, simply by making a few easy changes in your everyday life. So this section provides the know-how you need to reinforce the diet and exercise plan — without spending more than a very minimum of extra time. I've also a few suggestions as to what *not* to do in your quest for a flat stomach, in the hope that I can save you time, money and disappointment.

POSTURE

The most important thing you can do, not just for your stomach, but also for your shape and your looks from top to toe, is to learn how to stand, sit and move properly — what people call 'good posture'. Posture is such a pompous word — smacking of PE teachers at school and dance classes at the age of six — so that often the very word makes adults shudder. But if you can for a moment forget the 'books on head and ramrod-straight back' connection, all good posture means is carrying yourself about in a way that helps you feel good, look good, be efficient and balanced and is least likely to cause aches, pains and stress on joints and muscles.

Healthy new born babies don't have a posture problem — poor posture is learnt, gradually, throughout childhood and usually gets much much worse once we reach adulthood, so that eventually, sitting, standing and moving *wrongly* feels *right*. It's only when we look at our out-of-shape, out-of-line bodies in the mirror or wonder why our neck, shoulders, back, hips (etc, etc!) ache so much that it becomes a problem.

Poor posture is a vicious circle — after years of, say, standing wrongly, certain muscles will become overlong, others will become too short. Because muscles don't work in isolation, other parts of your body will mis-align themselves to try to compensate for the original imbalance and suddenly you've got not one problem, but two! And so on.

The single most common posture fault — to stand, sit and walk with the pelvis tipped forward and the small of the back in an exaggerated curve (Figure 52) — leads not only to a sticking-out stomach, but also to backache, tight hips, tight hamstrings, rounded shoulders, too-short chest muscles and a head that doesn't sit squarely on your shoulders but dips forward.

Once you decide to get your posture correct,

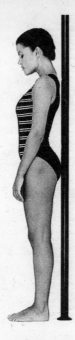

FIGURE 52

it will then take more than just deciding to — it will actually take conscious effort to get those muscles back as they were meant to be. This means following an exercise programme designed to correct the faults — and making a real effort every day to do things right.

The Flat Stomach Exercise Programme will help a great deal towards giving you good posture and the tips that follow will help even more. But if you have a severe problem it may be worth while doing extra exercises for your particular problem area. Stiffness is likely to be a major difficulty if your posture is very bad — so you could start with a beginners yoga or stretching course, perhaps, and add some strengthening exercises too.

Just as poor posture can be a downward spiral, once you begin to re-learn good posture, the upward spiral happens very quickly. The stomach exercises strengthen your stomach; this immediately gives more support to your back and pelvis so you soon begin to stand better too; the pelvic tilts also make standing better come more naturally; as you stand better your stomach gets even more used to sitting back in its right position and gets even stronger; hip muscles get looser as you begin to use your lower body correctly; your spine can now naturally stand straighter with less effort and so tension in shoulders and neck finally disappears.

To help this upward spiral along, here are three simple but very effective tips for you to remember, not just every day of your fifteen-day programme, but afterwards, too.

1. **Stand right**. Before you get dressed in the morning, do this simple exercise-cum-check to make sure you know how standing right really feels.

Stand with your back to the wall, a couple of inches away from the wall, hands at sides. Move backwards until your heels are about an inch from the wall. At this stage, your bottom and shoulders should touch the wall at the same time. If they don't, stand until they do. The back of your head should be virtually touching the wall, too. Now check your stomach — I bet it's sticking out! Your pelvis isn't tilted correctly, is it?! Tuck your bottom *in*, lift your pubic bone *up*, until your pelvis is aligned. You've got it right when your stomach miraculously 'disappears' (Figure 53).

Also make sure your chin is tucked in, not sticking out, that your shoulders are relaxed and down, not tense and hunched. If your shoulders are round you will need to pay particular attention to arm loosening exercises and upper back strengthening exercises before your posture will be perfect.

Stand there for a minute, getting used to the posture. Really think about how it feels — because this is the stance you should adopt all the time — when you're walking, too. Practise walking across the room, standing properly, now back again to the wall.

Now stretch your arms out to your sides and up above your head (Figure 54). Can you touch the wall above your head? Do this every morning and you'll help your waist slim down.

Remember — at first, standing properly may not feel right. That's because the 'right' muscles are underused, stiff, too short or too long. Keep at

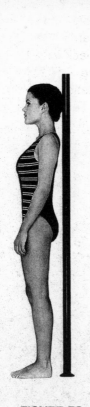

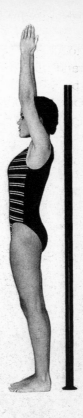

FIGURE 53   **FIGURE 54**

it and you'll soon have them as they should be!

Remember — standing right improves muscle tone all over your body *and* helps to flatten your stomach.

Repeat the wall exercise every morning and train yourself throughout every day to be aware of how you are standing.

Constantly wearing high heeled shoes is bad for your posture, too, as it tips you forward, so reserve heels higher than 1″ or so for special occasions and wear flatties as often as possible.

2. **Sit right**. If you're sitting now, reading this, *how* are you sitting? If you're in an easy chair, is your back firm against the back of the chair all the way down, or have you 'sunk'? If at a table or desk, are you curled up over the book with legs tucked beneath the chair or crossed?

Either of these positions contribute to the tummy-bulging, no-waisted shape of poor posture — and you've probably been sitting like that for *years*.

Some chairs are just made to make you sit badly — so resolve if you sit at a desk a lot, to get yourself a proper chair that supports your back.

The right way to sit is right back into the chair, with your pelvis tilted at the right angle so that your stomach moves in. Keep your legs uncrossed and if reading, bring the book up to reading level, rather than bending over to meet the book.

If you have to sit for long periods you will help to avoid shoulder and neck tension by adopting the right position — you can also help by doing a few arm-circles now and then, followed by a few arm lifts (reach for the ceiling first with one arm, then the other).

When watching TV you could from time to time lie on the floor instead and do a half body stretch or a few pelvic tilts. Every little helps!

3. **Be aware**. Good posture needs conscious effort at first. So as you go about your day's work, check yourself out now and then. As you go past shop windows or mirrors, take a look. As you stand in a queue waiting, check yourself out. Do a pelvic tilt. Relax your shoulders. Gradually your new posture will become habit, and gradually it will become as natural as your old posture was.

STOMACH STRENGTH

Work a few extra stomach strengthening movements into your daily routine and you'll see even better results than if you just do the exercise plan alone.

Don't just sit there! While you're sitting at work or watching TV, even travelling, you can use that time to help your stomach strength. There is one simple exercise that takes a minute to perform. You can do it several times in the day however busy you are.

Sit on the chair. (If at a desk, move the chair backwards first so that your knees can clear the edge of the desk.) Now grip the front edge of the chair, either side of your legs, with your hands (Figure 55) and simply lift legs together, with

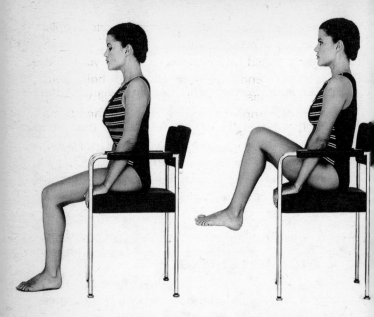

FIGURE 55   **FIGURE 56**

knees in the sitting position, towards your chest. Feel stomach muscles working to pull your legs up (Figure 56). Don't put too much pressure on hands. Hold the lift for a count of five then return legs slowly to floor. Repeat as many times as you can.

You'll also improve your stomach more quickly if you use it, and not your arms, to pull yourself out of the chairs and to slowly sink into chairs when you sit down. To do this all you need to remember is to avoid using your arms to help when you get up or sit down — if it sounds simple, try it and see what I mean!

Lastly, build more activities into your life. Many sports and weekend pursuits help your stomach muscles. Walking, especially hill walking, is ideal. It also improves your bottom line and firms up legs.

Swimming is perfect — it will help tremendously to improve your suppleness, your back mobility and strength, and your posture. Breast stroke is excellent for hip and shoulder mobility as well as stomach strength. Crawl is good for leg and bottom strength. But all swimming, if you do it regularly, will help you feel marvellous as well as look well toned and shapely.

Dancing, yoga and gymnastics are three other options for you to consider, though I wouldn't recommend taking up gymnastics if you're over a certain age!

When it comes to activity — do something you enjoy, otherwise you won't stick at it for long.

Think carefully before ...

Stomach-trimming gadgets of all kinds are one of the market leaders in the mail-order business. There are various kinds of gadgets — things you sit on and pull; things you sit on and push; things you stretch; things you kneel over and roll ... you name it. And I bet most of us have been tempted now and then to make a purchase. But will they really help you?

I am inclined to say that they won't. If you are already following the programme in this book these gadgets are unnecessary. Some of them — especially the roller kind that you push along the floor — can harm your back. Others exercise the wrong muscles because they don't 'isolate' your stomach muscles.

If you've been despairing of your stomach you may have wondered whether something as drastic as an operation is needed to get rid of belly bulge. You may have read case histories of people who have had *liposuction* — an operation that literally melts fat and sucks it out of your body. But, as I explained in Chapter 1, your fat stomach is very rarely caused by *fat* unless you are fat all over. And if you are fat all over, liposuction isn't recommended in any case. So that's not an option I would advise you to consider.

You may have heard of other people who have an *apronectomy* — an operation to remove loose skin from your stomach. Generally, people who have this operation are people who have been grossly overweight for years and their skin has lost its elasticity. In which case their GP recognises the problem and they have the operation performed on the NHS.

Some private clinics offer apronectomy. My view is that if you have really bad skinfolds that diet and exercise can't cure, then you should go to your GP. If you haven't, diet and exercise *will* cure the problem and so spending money on a private operation is a waste of your time and cash.

Your skin is much more flexible than you think — imagine how much it has to stretch in pregnancy. The muscles, too, under the skin are very, very adaptable. They will take a lot more stretching and neglect than you ever thought possible and still spring back into shape without any more drastic measure than diet, posture and exercise. Honestly!

CHAPTER SEVEN

Dress
to Impress

So now the diet, exercise plan and lifestyle tips have given you the flat stomach and neater, slimmer waist you always wanted — a better body altogether, in fact.

If you're very lucky, you may now have a *perfect* body — but to be honest, I doubt it. Very, very few people have perfectly-proportioned bodies in every respect, and that includes gymnasts, beauty queens, actresses and models. I can think of many top photographic and catwalk models who, while having lovely long legs, swan necks and slim hips, have no waist at all. The point is that they look lovely because they know how to make the best of themselves.

So if you have truly made the best of your body — bearing in mind that you can't alter your basic bone structure which gives you your figure *type*, stop worrying about minor imperfections — say, a waist that is 26″ when you really wanted it 24″, for example.

This chapter is devoted to making the best of your new figure — and making the world believe that it *is* perfect! And it's all down to what you choose to wear.

Some styles and fashions will make you look stunning; others will be neutral (neither improving your image nor detracting from it) while several styles will instantly make you look fatter, bigger or in one way or another stop you from looking your best.

And it's not just style that can have this effect — your choice of fabrics, materials, colours and accessories will do the same.

Even if you *do* have a perfect figure, by the way, do read on because although you may be able to wear anything and 'get away with it' that's not to say you should.

So for figure flattery, try these ideas for size. (There are tips for men in Chapter 9.)

BEFORE YOU SHOP

Before you even think of going near the stores to buy yourself something new, you should bear three very important points in mind. They can save you from making expensive mistakes — expensive both in terms of your self-confidence and your bank balance.

1. *Be honest about yourself.* Assess your best points and your not-so-good points. For instance, you may have good shoulders, a nice bustline, good arms, a fabulous waist, nice bottom, long legs, slim

ankles. On the minus side you may have a short neck, slightly large hips or unattractive knees. Make a list of your good and less good points and vow to buy to maximise the good and minimise the bad.

2. *Think of style, not fashion.* With the tips in this chapter and a little common sense, you can build up a selection of styles and looks that you know suit you. When you look for clothes, never forget that you should always go *first* for styles that suit you and then (and only then) should you go for what is in fashion at the moment. If what is 'in' this month or this season doesn't suit you, don't buy it. Don't be a fashion victim.

If you like high-quality clothes, buying the height of fashion which will be out of date in two or three months seems the quickest way to waste money. How will you get value out of it? If you're a student or teenager, low-cost, high-fun fashion is a good idea — but even then you should think of how things look on *you* first. The clever way to always be in fashion is to buy fashionable accessories instead — jewellery, shoes, belts, hats, scarves, bags can all instantly update an outfit without costing you a fortune.

3. *Trust your own opinion first.* Once you know what suits you, and what it is you're looking for on a particular shopping trip, don't let anyone else persuade you either into something you hadn't

intended to buy, or into something you're not sure suits you.

Sales assistants, however helpful they may be, are employed to sell, and won't be as impartial as you. Friends, daughters, husbands, mothers, all have different ideas of how you should look, and are probably also wondering how much longer you are going to be as, surely, it's time for lunch?

So you must learn to trust your own eye because *no one* is as interested in you as you are, *no one* knows your body as well as you do, and *no one* knows your tastes as well as you. To help *you* make the right decisions for *you*, here are a few more tips:

Go shopping alone.

Choose shops where you are left to browse in peace but where an assistant will help when asked, without interfering.

Take your time.

Don't shop when you're not 'in the mood'.

Don't shop for a specific event — say, a party — at the last minute.

LOOKS TO GO FOR — LOOKS TO AVOID

I've explained why the ultimate decision on an outfit must be yours, but here I've gathered together some specific advice on styles, fabrics, colours, patterns and accessories that will flatter your middle — and your figure altogether. And, just as important, I tell you what usually looks fattening or enlarging.

These are only guidelines and are drawn up specifically for people who are most concerned with minimising their stomach and waistline. For people with totally different figure concerns — say, overlarge hips or big legs, or people who are very short, or very tall — all the advice here may not apply, although much of it will.

Fabrics

Go for:

Linen, cotton, gabardines, fine wool, wool/polyester mixes; high quality acrylics, silks and fine jersey for suits, dresses, jackets, coats. For trousers, go for twill, cotton, denim, fine wool, crepe.

Avoid:

Fabrics that sag and bag — especially knits (for dresses and two-pieces); chiffon. Very rigid materials — such as canvas, tapestry. Overshiny-materials, such as satin. Very bulky fabrics, such as bouclé, chunky knits, thick corduroy, towelling.

Colours

It is more important to choose colours that suit your own skin, eyes, hair colouring and personality than to worry about which colours are fattening and which aren't. In fact, worn in the right styles and combinations, most colours are acceptable whatever your figure type.

Black. Now that you have made the best of your figure, there is no need to stick to black unless you are mad on it, although black *is* a slimming colour. If you like black, add touches of colour or white, or gold, to give interest. To make your waist look even smaller, the best 'black' trick I know is to go for a dress (or suit, swimsuit or leotard) which has black panels on the outside of your waist and a bright centre panel. If this mid-panel follows a concave curve to give you a 'false waist, even better!

White. People may tell you not to wear white unless you are a perfect size 10 — but you can. If the cut of the garment is good, the material non-bulky and non-clinging, but something that drapes gently, it can look very good. Particularly if you add one or two slimming touches — for instance, a deep V collar in a contrasting dark colour. But avoid white if you are very pale. Ivory and cream will suit you better.

Brights. Solid brights can be very slimming and flattering, as long as they suit your particular colouring.

Neutrals. These can be slimming, but can be dull too. Best on redheads and blondes or silver greys.

Gold, silver. You need a good figure to carry

off gold and silver lamé or lurex, especially if it is clingy, which it often is. All that shine — and sometimes bulk because of sequins and so on — adds inches. Go carefully.

Patterns

Patterned materials can be a wonderful style aid if you learn to use them to flatter you, and don't let them devour you.

All-over patterns. A patterned dress or suit, for instance. Match the size of pattern to your height — small women should avoid big patterns. Tall women can wear any size of pattern, but loud, big checks and horizontal stripes are the most fattening patterns; vertical stripes, small black and white checks, light dots on a dark background are the most slimming patterns.

Patterns mixed with plain. Remember attention will be drawn to the patterned section of your outfit — so make sure the pattern is on your good bits and the plain on your less good bits. For instance, if you want to minimise your waist, avoid a plain dress with a patterned belt or mid-section. If you are hippy, wear a patterned blouse tucked into a plain skirt — never a patterned jumper that finishes on the hip, or a patterned skirt with plain blouse tucked in.

STYLES

Dresses, skirts, suits

Flattering looks:
Small, soft shoulder pads to make waist look
smaller.
Tailored or unfussy dresses with simple lines and
minimum detail on body.
A-lines.
Knife pleats, stitched pleats falling from hip.
Culottes.
Wrapover dress with self belt and slight flare.
If you have slim legs — any V-shape, shift-type
dress with hemline narrower than shoulder line.
Add a medium or narrow belt if you have a small
waist.

Flattering accessories:
Dark belt with eyecatching buckle.
Belt dropped slightly below waist.
Belt worn comfortably loose.
On skirts, if you're short-waisted, a belt that
matches top, not skirt.

Fattening looks:
Anything gathered (dirndl). Avoid all gathered
styles unless you are reed-thin.
Circular skirts if you have anything less than a
perfect lower half.
Gored skirts, kilts.

Pleats of any kind that fall loose from the waist-band.

Skimpy cuts. Generously-cut clothes of the best quality you can afford always make you look slimmer than if you've squeezed into something small.

Belted, unstructured two-piece.

Short, straight cap sleeves.

Sleeves that end level with your waistline.

Straight skirt, unless you have a small waist and good legs

Tops

Flattering looks:

Boatneck, wide collar, shawl collar, cowlneck, peaked lapels, deep V-neck.

Gentle shoulder pads, yoke, epaulettes.

Set-in sleeves, Dolman sleeves.

Any shirt tailored to fit rather than left baggy.

Flared (not gathered) peplum — especially good for creating a small waist. Not so good for big hips or bottom.

Fattening looks:

Collars pointing or drooping towards the waist, crew neck.

Gathered peplum.

Belted tunic; chunky knit sweaters, cricket sweaters, sweatshirts.

Cap sleeves, puff sleeves.

Trousers, shorts, legwear

Flattering looks:

Leggings or footless tights underneath long, skinny sweater or T-shirt.

Jeans, straight-cut, plain or slightly pleated top, narrow belt, full-length leg.

Jumpsuits with dolman sleeve and narrow leather or elasticated belt.

Accessories:

Trousers always look good with heeled boots. Tuck jeans in.

Fattening looks:

All trousers or shorts with elasticated waistbands and/or gathers.

Jodhpur-styles.

Harem pants.

Very tapered leg (if you have big hips, big legs).

All styles that finish above the ankle — even worse if very wide-legged.

All tight waistbands that create a bulge over the top.

Towelling tracksuits.

Knitted trousers.

Coats and jackets

Flattering looks:

Tailored. Well-cut.

Single-breasted.

Cut-away to hip length.

Edge to edge.
Collarless over camisole top

Fattening looks:
Wrapover coats.
Fur or fake fur coats.
Padded, quilted jackets.
Tie-belt, unstructured coats ('the dressing-gown look').
Chanel jackets — short, boxy — unless you have a slim, long waist and neat hips and bottom.

Swimwear

Flattering looks:
All in ones. Stretchy, high Lycra content.
Lightly-formed cups.
Centre panel in brighter colour than outer panels.
Suit with racing stripe down outer edges.
Stripes going in a V from underarm to pubic bone.
High-cut legs.
V-neck racing suits.
Suits with broad shoulders and a deep V cutaway right down to mid-stomach.

Accessories:
Wide-brimmed hats to balance larger hips and thighs.
Big sunglasses, ditto. Beach wraps. Wedge sandals or shoes for longer legs. A light tan!

Fattening looks:
Bikinis — avoid unless you have perfect figure.

Twenties-look two-pieces. Those that cover you all
up except for a 1- or 2-inch gap at the waist.
Strapless bandeau tops.
Straight-across the top tops.
Towelling swimsuits.
Metallic finish.
Pure cotton.
Cut-out panels at either side of waist.

CHAPTER EIGHT

Baby Boom

Pregnancy is the most common cause of women losing their body tone and shape — not only while pregnant and in the weeks after the birth, but permanently. Only one in three mothers manage to get their pre-pregnancy shapes back completely. And if they have two, three, four or more children, the problem just gets worse and worse!

Yet it doesn't have to be that way. You *can* have children and make a complete return to your old shape after not just one baby — but after each baby.

Of course, it takes a little effort, but all the advice in this chapter that allows you to be a slim and flat-stomached mum weeks after the birth, will also help you to a healthier, fitter pregnancy and post-natal period. So do read on.

The secret is to watch your weight gain and your muscle tone during pregnancy, and follow a suitable diet and re-toning regime straight after the birth.

NOTE: This chapter is specifically for women from pre-conception to around three months after the birth, or whenever breastfeeding stops. If you have older children, you can follow the ordinary Flat

Stomach Diet (either maintenance or low-calorie) and Exercise Programme that appears in the earlier chapters.

IF YOU'RE THINKING OF HAVING A BABY

If you are planning on becoming pregnant soon, you need to be as fit, slim and healthy as you can before you conceive. You can follow the Flat Stomach Maintenance Diet and Exercise Programme if you don't need to lose any weight — both regimes are well-balanced and healthy, I assure you of that. If you need to lose some weight it is advisable to lose it before you become pregnant, as trying to lose your own body fat during pregnancy is fraught with problems and should only be done under supervision. If you do want to slim, then, follow the Flat Stomach Low-calorie Fifteen-day Diet in Chapter 3. And then make sure you read all of this chapter and start to carry out its advice the minute you know you're pregnant.

IF YOU'RE PREGNANT

The Flat Stomach 'Positive, Neutral, Negative' way of eating and, in early pregnancy, the Maintenance

Diet plan, are, in many ways, ideal for you if you are pregnant. However, pregnant women have fairly exact nutritional requirements and there are a few modifications you should make to the programme if you would like to follow it. I'll explain them now.

Diet in pregnancy

For a healthy baby — and a healthy you — you need a well-balanced, varied diet with lots of unrefined foods, fresh fruit and vegetables and plenty of protein, iron and calcium. The Flat Stomach Maintenance Diet should offer you sufficient quantities of most of all these nutrients during the first months of your pregnancy.

Protein: Pregnant women need more protein than usual — around 100 g a day. If following the Flat Stomach Diet, increase the daily skimmed milk allowance to 1 pint, or, for variety, replace any ¼ pint with one small pot of natural yogurt or real fruit yogurt. Other good sources of protein are lean meats and poultry, low-fat cheeses, and eggs.

Iron and vitamin C: In pregnancy many women become anaemic if they don't get enough iron. This is partly because a lot more blood is circulating when you're pregnant. Best sources of iron are liver and other offal, lean red meat, eggs, and leafy green vegetables.

Vitamin C helps absorption of iron in your body, so it's wise to eat or drink a C-rich item, such as oranges or orange juice, with iron-rich foods. Some foods — such as broccoli — contain both in one package and are therefore ideal. Vitamin C also helps keep your gums healthy while you're pregnant.

Calcium: Pregnant women need around 1,200 mg of calcium daily. The Flat Stomach Diet is rich in calcium and if you choose the calcium-rich choices when offered within the fifteen-day plan, you won't go short. Best calcium sources are milk, hard cheeses, yogurt, other cheeses and leafy vegetables.

Zinc: Many experts advise pregnant women to eat more zinc. Again, on the Flat Stomach Diet, you will get plenty, as good sources are certain nuts, hard cheese, sunflower seeds, oily fish and lean meat.

NOTE: You should avoid spinach (despite what you've heard about its iron content!) when you're pregnant, as well as cocoa and chocolate. These foods contain oxalic acid, which hinders your body's absorption of minerals. If following the Flat Stomach Diet, don't choose the spinach alternative where mentioned (Main Meal, Day 13; Main Meal, Day 14; Lunch, Day 15).

Salt: In pregnancy it is natural and normal to carry more body fluid, therefore, in order to retain the right salt/water balance within this fluid, you may need to get a little more salt into your diet, perhaps by adding a little more in cooking.

However, I wouldn't advise a high-salt diet — this could cause you to retain too much fluid and make your pregnancy uncomfortable.

The Flat Stomach Diet also helps you to a healthy pregnancy by being low in sugar and saturated fat. Importantly, it asks you to drink plenty of water, which is vital and it helps prevent the constipation that plagues so many pregnant women. And it asks you to eat 'little and often' — an excellent way of minimising sickness in early pregnancy and heartburn and indigestion in later pregnancy.

Eating for two

There is no need — unless you were too thin at the start of your pregnancy — to eat more than normal in the first five months or so. Just follow the guidelines above and eat *well*.

It is only in the last few months that you should increase your calorie intake — i.e, eat *more*. Even then, for women of average height and build, around 300 calories a day more is enough. These extra calories should also be in nutritious foods, low on saturated fat and sugar.

So I suggest that if you have been following the Flat Stomach Maintenance Programme in early pregnancy, around month FIVE you *add* these foods to your diet every day: two selections a day from List 1 and one selection a day from List 2 *plus* as much fruit and fresh vegetables as you feel like — don't stint on those.

List 1
2 oz/50 g lean red meat, liver or kidney
4 oz/100 g poultry or fish
1 oz/15 g hard cheese
1 small tub cottage cheese
1 large egg
1 small yogurt, plain or with fruit

List 2
4 oz/100 g potato, boiled or jacket
1 large slice wholemeal bread
1 oz/25 g wholegrain breakfast cereal
3 oz/75 g (cooked weight) brown rice
3 oz/75 g (cooked weight) wholewheat pasta

Weight gain in pregnancy
To remain too thin during pregnancy is positively dangerous — so don't even contemplate keeping your figure by using such a method. You should eat well and look forward to putting on 22+ lbs (10+ kgs).

On the other hand, too much weight gain can also be dangerous. It increases the risk of high blood pressure and of you suffering from backache, lethargy, varicose veins and a general feeling of being uncomfortable in the later stages. And too much weight gain makes it much harder to get your figure back after the birth.

So the most important thing you can do for your post-natal figure is to keep your weight under control while you are pregnant. That way, you won't be left with much *fat* to lose after the birth — and you'll minimise stretching of skin and, indeed, you'll help prevent stretchmarks.

Talking of stretchmarks, by the way — can you prevent them altogether? Many women do go through one — or several — pregnancies without getting a single stretchmark. Some of these women have deliberately done their best to avoid them; others have done nothing. So obviously part of the answer is that your own skin type, build and predisposition will decide whether you are going to get stretchmarks or whether you are not.

Certainly, if you stay within weight gain guide-lines, you will be doing the most sensible thing — obviously, the fatter you get, the more your skin will have to stretch and the more likely marks will be. But women who only put on 20lbs (9kgs) get stretchmarks, too — so that's not the whole answer.

Some women swear by rubbing oil into the abdomen every day while they are pregnant, and this may help by keeping your skin soft and supple — but again, there is no guarantee that any special cream or oil will prevent stretchmarks. *And*, by the way, you don't need to spend a fortune on expensive creams — baby oil will do just as well.

Lastly, if you can manage to minimise stretch-marks with the above tips, you will find they do fade after the birth and if you keep yourself in shape, with your skin in good condition, they will be barely noticeable.

I have read many different professional opinions on what the 'right' weight gain in pregnancy is — varying from 21 lbs (9.5 kgs) to 30 lbs (13.5 kgs) or more. My advice is that if you are small, you should aim to gain no more than 22 lbs (10 kgs). If you are tall and big boned, you could gain 28 lbs (12.5 kgs). Around 25 lbs (11.5 kgs), therefore, should be about right if you are 'average'. (Twins, by the way, usually come heavier!)

If you start putting on much more than this, the weight is inevitably going to be pounds of fat that definitely won't come rolling off after the baby is born without careful diet and exercise. As a guide, you should put on *no* weight in the first three months, then an average of 1 lb (450 g) a week or 4¼ lbs (2 kgs) a month after that.

If you start out at your right weight, it will be fairly easy to tell whether you're doing all right with a monthly weigh-in. Another way to keep a check is to measure the top of your thigh at the start of your pregnancy, then again once a month. If you are putting on inches — and therefore weight — there, it is excess fat rather than necessary weight.

If you start out overweight, you should ask your doctor or the dietician at the ante-natal clinic to advise you. In any case, you shouldn't follow a crash or very low-calorie diet to try to slim while you are pregnant. On such a diet you wouldn't be getting enough of the vital nutrients we've just talked about.

The lowest-calorie diet during pregnancy I have heard anyone recommend is 1,500 a day for women who are considered obese. Such a diet, carefully followed, should ensure no weight is gained or lost during the pregnancy so that in effect the mother has lost up to two stones of her own body fat while she was pregnant. However, I stress that your own doctor should decide whether or not you need to reduce calories while you are pregnant.

Exercise in pregnancy

If you want to get your figure back fast after the baby is born, you should keep your abdominal muscles toned up and keep yourself fit throughout the nine months. Though you can't avoid your stomach stretching as you grow larger (and who would want to when the 'bulge' is part of the fun!) you can keep those muscles elastic and strong so that they quickly return to normal.

Also your additional weight, your altered stance in later pregnancy, and the softer ligaments of pregnancy can all lead to the bane of the expect-ant mum — backache. Strong stomach muscles and some exercise can keep that at bay.

But hormonal changes in pregnancy and those soft ligaments mean that the kind of exer-cises you can do when you're not pregnant are sometimes best replaced by others when you are.

Particularly, you should avoid all straight-leg sit-ups and all exercises which require you to lift both legs into the air at once while lying down.

The Flat Stomach Exercise Programme is quite tough, and, unless you have been following it for a while so your stomach is already in good condition, you may prefer to do more gentle exercises once you are pregnant. In any case, I advise you to swop to the exercises that follow once you are into your last three months.

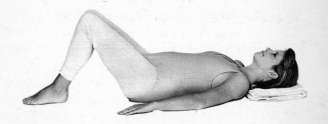

FIGURE 57

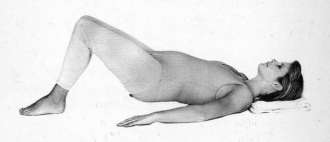

FIGURE 58

1. **A version of the pelvic tilt** (see Chapter 5).
    This is called the pelvic lift. Lie with your head
    on a small pillow, in pelvic tilt (Figure 57). Now,
    clenching your buttock muscles as tight as you
    can, and holding stomach in, lift your whole
    bottom and lower back area off the floor
    (Figure 58). Hold for 5; return to floor. Repeat
    as many times as you can manage without
    difficulty.

    In the last weeks of your pregnancy you
    can simply do the ordinary pelvic tilt.
2. **A version of the knees-in** (see Chapter 5).
    Lie in same position above. Do a pelvic tilt.
    Now, maintaining the tilt, slowly slide your feet
    forward until your legs are flat on the floor.
    Now slide left leg back and bring it in towards
    your body as in the knees-in (Figures 59 & 60).
    In the later stages of pregnancy, you won't be
    able to bring your knees in far at all!

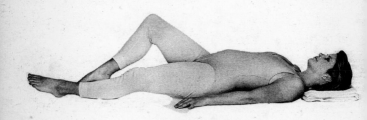

FIGURE 59

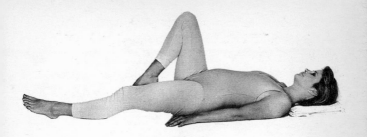

FIGURE 60

3. **The pelvic lift**, version 2.
Some women may find this more comfortable, especially in late pregnancy, than exercise 1. If you're feeling fine, you could do both. Find a small sturdy stool, preferably upholstered for your comfort. Lie on floor with head on cushion, arms at sides. Now put your feet on the stool, keeping legs straight. Do a pelvic tilt, tightening stomach and buttock muscles as much as you can (if you can't feel your stomach

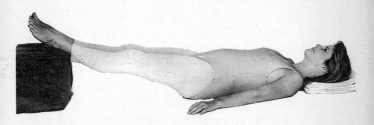

FIGURE 61

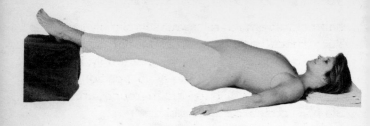

FIGURE 62

muscles in late pregnancy, concentrate on your bottom instead) (Figure 61). Now simply raise your bottom off the floor, count to five and lower (Figure 62). Do five or more if you can manage it.

Posture

Good posture is vital throughout your pregnancy. It helps prevent backache and keeps stomach muscles strong. So read all the advice in Chapter 6 relating to posture. As the weight on your stomach increases, you may find yourself adopting a stance where your upper body sways back to compensate. Try to avoid this by keeping your lower back flat, and don't wear high heels.

Stretching

Because your ligaments are soft and over-stretching could cause sprains and strains, it is best to avoid the long body stretch and other stretching exercises while you are pregnant. But you can do a half-body stretch to relax yourself. Simply lie on the floor, knees bent, head on small flat cushion and arms above head. Lie, breathing naturally, for a few minutes. If the 'arms above head' position feels at all uncomfortable, bring them round and down until you do feel comfortable.

You can also do a wall stretch. Sit with back against a wall, and lift first one arm and then the other high above you until you touch the wall. Keep the pelvis aligned properly throughout this exercise (Figure 63).

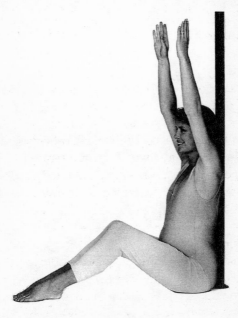

FIGURE 63

Sports and activities

To keep yourself fit — and help your stomach and back muscles — a little exercise every day is a good idea. Swimming is perfect, especially in the later stages of pregnancy when the water will carry your weight. Walking is good, too. Dangerous activities such as riding and skiing should be avoided.

Exercise will help prevent circulation problems and varicose veins.

NOTE: Anyone with complications in pregnancy and/or a history of miscarriage should get her doctor's or ante-natal clinic's advice before beginning or continuing any exercise programme.

AFTER THE BIRTH

Your diet

If you've followed all the advice in this chapter, you should be near your normal weight a week or two after the birth.

If you are breastfeeding

Breastfeeding is a good idea, not only for the obvious reasons that it's good for baby and convenient, but also because it actually helps your uterus (womb) shrink quickly back to its normal size, and it uses up around an extra 500 calories a day, so if you do have a few pounds to lose you won't find it a problem.

In that case, I suggest you follow the Maintenance Flat Stomach Diet plan *plus* an extra 500 calories a day of healthy foods and drinks — lean proteins, fruit, vegetables, milk. The Positive, Neutral, Negative way of eating is very suitable for breastfeeding mothers — but do drink plenty of liquid.

Here are two examples of foods adding up to 500 calories that you could add to the Maintenance Flat Stomach Plan:

Example 1

½ pint/300 ml skimmed milk
2 oz/50 g Edam cheese and salad
1 medium slice wholemeal bread with low-fat
    spread
½ oz/15 g sunflower seeds or 2 oz/50 g lean
    chicken

Example 2

1 natural yogurt and chopped fruit
1 oz/25 g almonds or unsalted peanuts
1 small tub cottage cheese
3 rye crispbreads with low-fat spread

You can either take these extras as separate snacks, or add them to a meal.

Or you could simply increase calories by increasing the portion sizes on the Flat Stomach Diet. The calorie chart in Chapter 10 will help you easily to add the right amount of the foods you choose.

If you aren't breastfeeding
You can simply follow the Maintenance Diet in Chapter 3, or build your own diet of around 2,000 calories a day using the Positive, Neutral, Negative food listings in Chapter 2 and the calorie chart in Chapter 10.

However, if you ARE overweight ...

If you have more than a few pounds to lose, here's what you should do:

If you are breastfeeding
You should follow the Maintenance Plan in Chapter 3, making sure to drink plenty of the 'unlimited' liquids, plus all your skimmed milk and other liquids mentioned in the diet.

Because the Maintenance Plan doesn't allow for the extra 500 calories you will be using up by breastfeeding, you will build up a weekly calorie 'deficit' of 3,500, on which you should lose at least 1 lb (450 g) a week, perhaps more at first. This may not sound much, but you really mustn't try to crash diet when breastfeeding.

Once you reach your correct weight, if you are still breastfeeding, follow the plan above for breastfeeding mothers who don't need to lose weight.

If you aren't breastfeeding
You can start on the Flat Stomach Weight Loss

Diet in Chapter 3. This is a healthy balanced diet of around 1,200 calories a day and will help keep your energy levels up while you lose 1-2 lbs (450 g-900 g) a week (more at first). By following the Flat Stomach Positive, Neutral, Negative theory you will help your stomach return to normal as quickly as possible.

Getting back in shape

After the birth, unless you had particular problems, you can begin to exercise almost straight away — but you must take it easy at first. Use the advice that follows and you should have your flat stomach back within two to three months. Some women do it in four to six weeks!

Days 1 and 2 after the birth
You can begin stomach exercises while lying on your bed. The best ones are the ante-natal exercises you learnt earlier in this chapter (see page 168). If they cause you any pain, stop and try again tomorrow. But everyone should be able to do several pelvic tilts without trouble. Practise holding your stomach muscles *in* while you do the pelvic tilt.

Do them as many times in a day as you can manage.

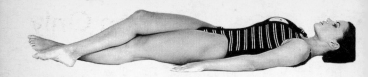

FIGURE 64

Days 3-7
Do the following exercises from Chapter 5:
The warm-ups (see pages 105-110).
The Pelvic Tilt (see page 102).
Exercise One — the Curl-Up (Grade 1) (see page 111).
Exercise Two — the Crossed Curl (Grade 1) (see page 114).
PLUS this new exercise: The Leg Cross. Lie, arms at sides, and simply bring your right leg over your left leg to touch the floor (or bed) beyond your left leg (Figure 64). Hold for 5. Repeat other side.

Days 7-14
Do the exercises as days 3-7, but ADD:
Exercise Five — Diagonal Lifts (Grade 1) (see page 121).

Week 2 onwards
Do the complete Flat Stomach Exercise Programme, staying on Stage 1 with every exercise until your post-natal six-week check. Then continue with the Programme, building up to Stage 3 according to your own progress.

CHAPTER NINE

Men Only

So you have finally decided that your spare tyre isn't stunning, your beer belly isn't beautiful and that you really *must* do something about it. Congratulations.

Don't let anyone, in that case, accuse you of being vain. Because if you do slim down your stomach, you'll be doing your health a very big favour too.

Here's why.

While women naturally tend to carry surplus fat on their hips and thighs and only to a lesser extent across their stomachs (see 'Is it fat?', Chapter 1), men frequently carry extra weight in the area between chest and hips. And studies show that if most of your surplus weight is on your middle body rather than in other areas, such as your legs or on your chest, you are more likely to suffer from heart disease (and, incidentally, diabetes). This 'apple shape' theory ties in well with the fact that men are more prone to heart trouble than women are.

So if you are a typical 'apple' male, with slim arms and legs, not far off your right weight for height (see chart on page 183), but with a waist and stomach you're always trying to hide — don't delay. Now is the time to get yourself in shape. With a straightforward programme of the right diet and exercise you can do it easily.

BEER BELLIES — FACT AND FICTION

You have a 'beer belly'? Here's some news. There is *nothing* special in the beer that you drink which causes it to 'stay on your stomach' — apart from the calories it contains!

Ordinary beer contains 200 calories a pint, strong beers can go up to 400 — so you can see how, if you're a five-pints-a-night man, those pints can easily convert to fat. However, the same is true of any food if you eat more than you need. Should you be prone to overeating on chocolate, or Chinese, or chips, the result would be the same. You'll put on weight — and if, like many men, you're a natural 'apple', the weight will go on your middle.

As men seem more partial to a pint than a packet of sweets, hence the myth of the beer belly. And *your* beer belly (whatever caused it!) can be beaten, I can assure you, with the Flat Stomach Diet and Exercise Plan. And having said that, I shall now qualify myself by adding that some men do find that beer gives them a 'gassy stomach' so their bellies swell up with wind in the few hours after drinking it.

If you like beer and that's your problem, try switching to a different brand or type — for instance, Guinness is often a culprit, and real ale often suits men who can't take ordinary brews.

If you are one of those men who gets 'blown up' on *all* beer — well, how about a nice glass of wine?!

THE FLAT STOMACH DIET — PERFECT FOR YOU

The Flat Stomach Eating Plan is ideal for all men with a big belly or spare tyre. Not only will it help you lose that flab *fast*, it also ties in perfectly with all the latest research findings on diet and heart disease. It will also improve your digestion and your skin, it will keep your energy levels high and prevent hunger while you trim down.

The diet is:

- Low in saturated fat and cholesterol. The total fat level is well within official UK guidelines. However, the diet contains a good balance of mono- and poly-unsaturated fats including Omega-3s (the 'good for you' kinds).
- Low in salt. Too much salt aggravates high blood pressure and can, some experts believe, *lead* to high blood pressure and an increased risk of heart disease and stroke.
- High in beta-carotene (a substance found in green, yellow and orange vegetables and certain fruits), and in vitamins E and C — all

three are 'anti-oxidant' vitamins. Different research studies have shown a link between low levels of these anti-oxidants and high levels of heart disease, and a link between a high intake of them and a reduced risk of heart disease — and cancer, too.

The Flat Stomach Diet is also low in sugar and high in soluble fibres (now thought more beneficial than the wheat-based insoluble fibres).

However, it isn't an unpalatable diet. Spices, red meats (if you want them), butter, cheese and eggs are all allowed. Even beer or other alcohol is allowed in moderation if you are following the Maintenance Plan.

The diet is based on a high intake of POSITIVE foods, an adequate intake of NEUTRAL foods, and avoidance, as far as possible, of NEGATIVE foods. For a more detailed explanation of the POSITIVE/ NEUTRAL/NEGATIVE theory and system of eating which literally flattens your stomach while you eat and drink, read Chapter 2.

Now, just decide which of the following regimes would most suit you, then you can start.

Are you at, or near, your correct weight?

Take your clothes off and look in the mirror. If most of your body seems to be fine but you just have a small 'pot' and/or some surplus flab around your middle, you probably don't need to go on a low-calorie diet. If you're not certain, check your weight against the height/weight chart here. If you're near average for your height, I suggest you follow the Maintenance Diet for men which appears below.

HEIGHT/WEIGHT CHART FOR MEN

Height	Average weight	Acceptable weight range
5ft 4ins 1.62 metres	130lbs 59kgs	118-148lbs 53.5-67kgs
5ft 5ins 1.65 metres	133lbs 60.5kgs	121-152lbs 55-69kgs
5ft 6ins 1.67 metres	136lbs 62kgs	124-156lbs 56.5-71kgs
5ft 7ins 1.70 metres	140lbs 63.5kgs	128-161lbs 58-73kgs
5ft 8ins 1.73 metres	145lbs 66kgs	132-166lbs 60-75.5kgs
5ft 9ins 1.75 metres	149lbs 68kgs	136-170lbs 62-77kgs
5ft 10ins 1.78 metres	153lbs 69.5kgs	140-174lbs 63.5-79kgs
5ft 11ins 1.80 metres	158lbs 72kgs	144-179lbs 65.5-81kgs
6ft 0ins 1.83 metres	162lbs 73.5kgs	148-184lbs 67-84kgs
6ft 1in 1.85 metres	166lbs 75.5kgs	152-189lbs 69-86kgs
6ft 2ins 1.88 metres	171lbs 78kgs	156-194lbs 71-88kgs
6ft 3ins 1.90 metres	176lbs 80kgs	160-199lbs 73-90kgs
6ft 4ins 1.93 metres	181lbs 82kgs	164-204lbs 75-93kgs

The combination of special foods, plus the exercise plan, will be enough to get your stomach into shape.

Alternatively you can use the listings in Chapter 2 plus the calorie chart in the next chapter to devise your own diet on a longer-term basis.

Are you overweight?

If you are at the upper end of the 'acceptable' weight range given for your height, or over it, you need to lose some weight. I suggest you follow the fifteen-day plan in Chapter 3, using the figures in brackets. These figures are a maintenance diet for women, but will produce a steady weight loss in men. Depending on your starting weight, you could lose up to 10 lbs (4.5 kg) in the fifteen days. That, coupled with your exercise plan, is all you need for a flat stomach. Please read all of Chapter 2 before you begin.

Once you have reached your ideal weight, switch to the Maintenance Plan below.

THE MALE MAINTENANCE DIET

Instructions
You eat five times a day — a breakfast, two portable snacks, a portable lunch, and an evening meal. You can have the evening meal at lunchtime if you

prefer. If you or your partner like to cook, there are recipe alternatives for one meal a day which appear in Chapter 4.

Don't add salt to your meals at table — you'll very soon get used to the 'real' flavour of food and soon oversalted food will taste awful. But you can use a salt substitute (such as LoSalt) if you like, or cut down salt little by little over a few days.

VEGETARIANS can follow the diet, too, just by swopping any meals you can't eat with the suggestions given at the end of each day.

UNLIMITED

All these are unlimited on the diet: fresh and dried herbs, lemon juice, salad leaves of any kind, herb teas, fruit teas, water and mineral water.

DRINKS

You have a daily allowance of half a pint skimmed or semi-skimmed milk for use in tea and coffee or on its own. Limit your use of tea and coffee to a couple of cups a day. Other milk mentioned in the diet is extra to this.

Drink as many herbal and fruit teas as you like, and have plenty of water — a glass with every meal is ideal.

Beer and other alcohol

Because, as I explained earlier, there is nothing specific about beer that gives you a pot belly, you can still drink it in moderation *and* get or keep a flat stomach. What matters is that you don't consume — in food or drink — more calories a day than you need.

Therefore, on the Maintenance Plan only, I've set aside 200 calories a day maximum for beer or other alcohol. So in addition to all the foods and drinks listed above and in the diet, you can have *per week* (to use as and when you like):
EITHER 7 pints beer or lager (not strong)
OR 7 large scotches or other spirits plus low-calorie mixers
OR 14 glasses wine.
These figures are *maximum* — if you don't want to use your drinks allowance, simply substitute 200 calories' worth of any other POSITIVE or NEUTRAL food using the calorie charts in the next chapter.

DAY 1

On rising
Cup lemon tea

Breakfast
7 fl oz (⅓ pint) glass orange juice

7 fl oz (⅓ pint) bowl Greek strained yogurt with 1 banana chopped in
1 medium slice wholemeal or oatbran bread with sunflower spread and 2 teaspoons honey or reduced-sugar marmalade

Snack
2 rye crispbreads with 4 oz/100 g cottage cheese

Lunch
3 oz/75 g Brie on 2 rye crispbreads with sunflower spread
Mixed salad of tomato, lettuce (any type), watercress, red pepper, cucumber and chopped basil, tossed in French dressing or with 1 dessertspoon mayonnaise
1 peach or apple

Snack
2 oz/50 g sunflower seeds
Cup herb tea

Main Meal
Large portion grilled, baked or microwaved chicken
6 oz/175 g potatoes
Salad of 1 stick celery, chopped, ½ apple, 1 oz/25 g walnut pieces, all mixed in 1 dessertspoon reduced-calorie mayonnaise and 1 dessertspoon natural yogurt mixed with 1 teaspoon lemon juice; chopped parsley

OR
1 portion Saffron Chicken with double portion
Orange Rice (see recipe page 68)
OR
1 portion Honeyed Chicken (see recipe page 70)
plus 8 tablespoons brown rice
8 oz/225 g slice melon plus 4 oz/100 g vanilla ice-
cream with any selection

Vegetarian suggestion: large baked potato filled
with large portion dahl (lentil purée) plus celery
and apple side salad as before.

DAY 2

On rising
Fruit tea, any variety

Breakfast
A mixed fresh fruit salad of melon, strawberries or
kiwifruit, pineapple, apple and banana with 4 oz/
100 g natural fromage frais and 1 teaspoon honey;
½ oz/15 g 'no added sugar' muesli on top
1 medium slice wholemeal bread with sunflower
spread and 1 teaspoon honey

Snack
2 ricecakes or 1 oatcake with 1 tablespoon peanut
butter

Lunch
Salad as Day 1
1 small whole ripe avocado, filled with French dressing
1 large slice wholemeal bread with sunflower spread

Snack
1 thick and creamy fruit yogurt
3 oz/75 g 'no need to soak' dried apricots

Main Meal
10 oz/275 g fillet white fish, any variety, baked, grilled or microwaved
8 oz/225 g jacket potato with ½ oz/15 g butter
6 oz/175 g broccoli
4 oz/100 g whole beans
Lemon to garnish
OR
1 portion Italian Fish Steaks (see recipe page 70)
OR
1 portion Sole in Mushroom Sauce (see recipe page 71) plus vegetables as above
4 oz/100 g grapes, 1 banana and 1 oz/25 g Brie with any selection

Vegetarian suggestion: omit fish and add 2 oz/50 g flaked toasted almonds to the vegetables before serving. Add extra ounce Brie to dessert.

DAY 3

On rising
Lemon tea

Breakfast
Whole grapefruit
3 oz/75 g 'no added sugar and salt' muesli with ¼ pint/150 ml skimmed or semi-skimmed milk
1 medium slice wholemeal or oatbran bread with sunflower spread and honey or reduced-sugar marmalade

Snack
4 oz/100 g skimmed milk soft or cottage cheese
2 sticks celery and 5 dates

Lunch
2 hard-boiled eggs, halved, on bed of lettuce and covered with 1½ tablespoons reduced-calorie mayonnaise
Watercress or parsley to garnish
1 large slice wholemeal bread with sunflower margarine
1 orange, 1 banana

Snack
2 oz/50 g shelled hazelnuts
5 fl oz/150 ml natural yogurt

Main Meal
2 medium extra-lean trimmed lamb chops, grilled
4 oz/100 g peas or mangetout
6 oz/175 g carrots or leeks, lightly cooked
6 oz/175 g low-salt instant mashed potato or 6 oz/
175 g baked potato
2 teaspoons mint sauce
¼/10 g butter
OR
1 portion Moroccan Lamb (see recipe page 72)
with 7 tablespoons boiled brown rice
OR
1 portion Braised Citrus Beef (see recipe page 73)
plus large portion spring greens and 6 oz/175 g
new potatoes
4 oz/100 g cherries plus 1 apple with any selection

Vegetarian suggestion: serve 2 × 4 oz/100 g Vege-
Burgers instead of the lamb.

DAY 4

On rising
7 fl oz (⅓ pint) orange juice

Breakfast
2 oz/50 g 'no need to soak' dried apricots, chopped
and stirred into 6 oz/175 g Greek strained yogurt
1 banana

Snack
1 apple
2 rice cakes or 1 oatcake topped with 4 oz/100 g skimmed milk soft cheese and cucumber

Lunch
8 oz/225 g slice melon
5 oz/150 g cooked chicken, lean only
Cucumber and tomato salad with chopped basil
1 large wholemeal roll with sunflower spread
OR
1 portion Chicken, Rice and Beansprout Salad (see recipe page 73)
plus ½ oz/15 g almonds

Snack
1 orange
1 oz/25 g sunflower seeds

Main Meal
½ grapefruit
6 oz/175 g salmon steak or fillet
OR
10 oz/275 g trout on bone, baked, poached or microwaved
OR
1 portion Fennel Trout (see recipe page 74)
4 oz/100 g mangetout or green beans
8 oz/225 g new potatoes with ¼ oz/10 g butter
Lemon to garnish

4 oz/100 g soft fruit of choice with 1 fl oz/25 ml Elmlea or single non-dairy cream

Vegetarian suggestion: use 5 oz/150 g diced tofu in your lunchtime salad; 1 large nut cutlet instead of fish.

DAY 5

On rising
Lemon tea

Breakfast
1½ oz/35 g any wholegrain, low-salt breakfast cereal, e.g. Shredded Wheat or Weetabix, with skimmed or semi-skimmed milk to cover
1 medium slice wholemeal or oatbran bread with sunflower spread and honey or reduced-sugar marmalade
1 apple

Snack
8 oz/225 g slice melon or 1 orange
2 oz/50 g Edam cheese and 2 rye crispbreads

Lunch
A salad of 4 oz/100 g tuna in oil, well drained and mixed with chopped cucumber, celery, apple and 5 oz/150 g cooked weight wholewheat pasta, all

tossed in French dressing and served on a bed of salad leaves garnished with chopped parsley

Snack
Slice melon
1 Petit Fromage Frais with Fruit
½ pint/300 ml semi-skimmed milk

Main Meal
1 large breast of chicken portion, skinned and covered with a paste of 2 fl oz/50 ml natural low-fat yogurt mixed with 1 tablespoon tandoori powder and grilled over medium heat for 30 minutes or baked for 45 minutes
8 oz/225 g boiled brown rice
2 tablespoons chopped cucumber and natural yogurt
1 tomato, sliced and garnished with chopped basil
½ chapati
OR
1 portion Chicken Paprika (see recipe on page 75)
OR
Sherried Turkey (see recipe page 76) served with 8 oz/225 g new potatoes and a green side salad with French dressing
3 oz/75 g ice-cream with any selection

Vegetarian suggestion: use 3 oz/75 g Mozzarella cheese in the lunchtime salad; have 1 large baked aubergine in the evening, sprinkled with

1½oz/35g toasted sesame seeds, plus the rice and side dishes.

DAY 6

On rising
7 fl oz (⅓ pint) orange juice

Breakfast
6 fl oz/175 ml natural yogurt topped with 6 oz/175 g strawberries, raspberries or sliced kiwifruit, plus ½oz/15g oatflakes
1 medium slice wholemeal or oatbran bread with sunflower spread and honey or reduced-sugar marmalade

Snack
2 rye crispbreads with 1 tablespoon peanut butter

Lunch
Slice melon
A salad of 2½oz/65g hazelnuts or unsalted peanuts mixed with 6oz/175g carrot, grated, and 2oz/50g dates, chopped, plus 1 teaspoon anise seeds (optional), all tossed in a dressing of 1 tablespoon olive oil mixed with 2 fl oz/50 ml orange juice, pepper and a little salt substitute
1 pitta bread

Snack
1 orange and 1 banana
1 fromage frais with fruit

Main Meal
6 oz/175 g extra lean roast beef
6 oz/175 g new potatoes
5 oz/150 g cauliflower
5 oz/150 g spring greens
4 oz/100 g swede, puréed
1 dessertspoon home-made horseradish sauce
Gravy made from beef juices and a little beef stock
thickened with 1 teaspoon cornflour
OR
1 portion Stir-Fried Beef with Oyster Sauce (see
recipe page 76)
PLUS 4 oz/100 g boiled brown rice or noodles
OR
1 portion Mushroom Pilau (see recipe page 77)

DAY 7

On rising
Fruit tea, any variety

Breakfast
½ grapefruit
1 boiled egg
2 medium slices wholemeal bread with sunflower

spread; 2 teaspoons honey
1 banana

Snack
1 peach or nectarine
1 Petit Fromage Frais with Fruit

Lunch
4 oz/100 g Mozzarella, sliced
3 medium tomatoes, sliced
Chopped basil
1 tablespoon olive oil
Leaf salad of choice
Large slice wholemeal bread with sunflower spread

Snack
2 rye crispbreads with 1 tablespoon peanut butter
1 orange

Main Meal
6 oz/175 g lean fillet or rump steak, grilled
6 oz/175 g new potatoes
5 oz/150 g broccoli
4 oz/100 g peas
1 medium tomato
Little gravy from stock cube
OR
1 portion Mustard Steak (see recipe page 91) served with 4 oz/100 g new potatoes, 5 oz/150 g broccoli and 1 tomato

OR
1 portion Lentil Bolognese with Pasta (see recipe page 92)

DAY 8

On rising
Fruit tea, any variety

Breakfast
6oz/175g Greek strained yogurt with 8oz/225g mixed fruit, chopped, and 1 teaspoon honey; topped with 1oz/25g 'no added sugar or salt' muesli

Snack
1 banana
2oz/50g 'no need to soak' apricots

Lunch
2 rye crispbreads with sunflower spread
4oz/100g cubed Edam cheese combined with 6oz/175g cubed melon, 1 ring fresh (or canned in natural juice) pineapple, cubed, 2oz/50g cucumber, diced, and all tossed in lemon juice with pinch ground ginger, 1 dessertspoon olive oil and chopped parsley to garnish

Snack
1 orange
1 fruit yogurt

Main Meal
10 oz/275 g fillet of monkfish or cod, baked in foil or microwaved
5 oz/150 g sliced green peppers and 5 oz/150 g sliced tomato, stir-fried in a non-stick pan in 1 dessertspoon corn or rapeseed oil
6 oz/175 g boiled brown rice or jacket potato
OR
1 portion Monkfish Kebabs (see recipe page 80), served with 7 tablespoons boiled brown rice

Vegetarian suggestion: par-boil 1 cubed aubergine, brush with corn oil and use on kebabs instead of the fish in recipe.

Days 9-15 — repeat Days 1-7.

THE FLAT STOMACH EXERCISE PLAN

The Exercise Programme in Chapter 5 is just as suitable for men as it is for women, so if you want a flat stomach — and an end to the 'saddlebag' look of a flabby waistline — start the programme now. It is fine for all levels of fitness as you progress at your own pace — but check with your doctor first if you are not in normal health.

After you've reached Grade 3, you may like to add wrist and ankle weights to the stomach exercises 1-6 to make them a little more difficult.

Once your stomach is as flat as you would

like it to be, all you have to do then is a complete programme twice a week to maintain your new look.

Get active!

Now you're getting yourself into shape, you should consider building more activity into your life so that you become aerobically fit too — in other words, you have more stamina. Many men do a good deal of sport when they are students. They also cycle because they can't afford a car — or walk. They go out dancing, and generally keep very fit. But in your twenties and thirties, it is so easy to let all that go. No more school, no more college. Car comes along, fitness disappears.

To be aerobically fit is not only good for your heart — it helps burn off calories that would otherwise settle on your waistline.

So do something from the list that follows every day — it doesn't always have to be the same thing. Do a minimum of twenty minutes, and build up slowly. You should also restart team games you used to enjoy once you get fitter.

- Walking. Walk as briskly as you can without feeling totally out of breath. Add hill walking for harder work.
- Cycling. Build up speed and distance gradually — again, add hill work later.
- Jogging. Progress to jogging, if you like, from

walking. But try to stay off hard road surfaces and wear good cushioning shoes.

- Swimming. Any stroke will do, but keep going! Remember, that's not always easy in a crowded pool.

CLOTHESWISE

The way that you dress can help you look better, whether you're still trying to disguise that belly or whether you're now slim. Here are some hints to help you.

Disguises while you're getting there

Trousers with a too-tight waistband under your 'pot' are never going to look any good. Neither are shirts straining at the buttons over the bulge. Nor is any belt that goes across or under the fat belly — it just draws the eye right to your worst area. So avoid, like the plague, all three of these mistakes.

Always wear a slightly loose waistband, and bear in mind these points:

- Suits (casual for weekend or the classic suit) always look better than trousers and shirt or sweater.
- The ideal suit style is Armani — wide-shouldered, slightly unstructured without being

too baggy, slightly tapered look from top to toe. Very flattering.

- A waistcoat will cover and minimise a fat middle.
- Single or double breasted suits can both look good depending on the cut of the individual suit — buy the best cut and the best cloth you can afford.
- Forget short or cropped jackets — hip length is much more flattering.
- For casual wear, forget all vest tops and T-shirts that cling, all crew-necked jumpers, especially if they are close fitting around the shoulders, all chunky knits. Go for big T-shirts to hip level and if you wear a sweater, have it in fine material with a loose raglan sleeve, and wear it over a shirt with an open-necked collar.
- Go for one size larger in your sweater than you think you need.
- Avoid velour and sweatshirt fabrics.

Now you're slim

Make yourself look even slimmer:

- Still bear in mind all the above tips.
- Never wear clothes that are too small. A 'just skimming' line makes you look twice as slim.
- Vertical lines running up the sides of trousers or tracksuit look good.
- Sweaters with a V or vertical pattern or line to

them somewhere look good.

- Pleated trousers hang better than flat-fronted trousers.
- Low-waisted trousers can make you look longer in the body and give you a narrower waistline.
- Avoid flares unless you have very long, slim legs.

CHAPTER TEN

Now Keep That Stomach Flat

Your fifteen-day programme of diet and exercise is finished — and you want to know what to do now.

Right. First, take a good look at yourself and your new shape in the mirror. The fifteen-day plan is long enough for most people, with 'average' problem tums and not more than 7-10 lbs (3-4.5 kg) to lose. Most of you will therefore be 100% happy with your new looks. But if you were very overweight, or if you had an extremely fat stomach, maybe you will decide that there is still room for further improvement. In that case, you can stay on the complete forty-minute workout — perhaps coupled with the low-calorie diet — a little longer. In fact, you can stay on it as long as you need, until you're exactly the shape you want to be.

Otherwise, all you have to do is complete the exercise programme in Chapter 5 a maximum of TWICE A WEEK to keep your stomach flat in the future. It's best to stay with a high grade rather than down-grading. By now the routine will probably take you only thirty minutes each time.

If you ever find yourself very busy it is better to do a short version of the programme than nothing at all. This should take a maximum of twenty minutes — hardly a lot to ask, is it? But think very carefully before saying 'I'm too busy.' The twice-weekly routine should be a habit you enjoy and look forward to and you should give yourself this personal time every week. What is more important than keeping yourself in shape?

The short programme is as follows:

WARM UPS as before. Don't skip these.
Exercise 2 — The Crossed Curl
Exercise 3 — Curl Back
Exercise 6 — The Crunch
Exercise 8 — Cobra and Child
Exercise 10 — The Lunge
COOL DOWN — Long Body Stretch of three minutes

Do your pelvic tilt before Exercises 2, 3, and 6 and your knees-in afterwards.

The twice-weekly routine, plus as much other activity as you can fit into your life — walking, swimming, cycling or whatever you choose — will keep you all-round fit. And don't forget the posture pointers in Chapter 6. They are very important. If you don't maintain good posture you won't maintain a flat stomach!

Your diet
You have your Maintenance Plan as detailed in

Chapter 3 (women) or Chapter 9 (men). This is suitable for as long as you care to use it, but for long-term I suggest you devise some snacks and meals of your own, using the calorie charts that follow and the POSITIVE/NEUTRAL listings in Chapter 2.

The POSITIVE/NEUTRAL/NEGATIVE theory is a *healthy* way to eat for always.

> Why not write and let me know how YOU got on on the Flat Stomach Diet and Exercise Plan? I'd love to hear from you. Write to me, Judith Wills, c/o Sphere Books, Orbit House, 1 New Fetter Lane, London EC4A 1AR.

CALORIE GUIDE

The following chart lists all the major POSITIVE and NEUTRAL foods you will be eating on the Flat Stomach Diet.
All calories are approximate.

Breads and crispbreads

Granary bread, per oz/25 g	70
Oatbran bread, per oz/25 g	65
Rye bread, black, per oz/25 g	90
Rye bread, light, per oz/25 g	70
Wholemeal bread, per oz/25 g	60
Wholewheat pitta bread, large, per item	170
Wholewheat pitta, mini, per item	90
Wheatgerm, e.g. Hovis, per oz/25 g	65
Oatcake, per cake	50
Rice cake, per cake	25

Rye crispbreads, per item:

Finn Crisp	40
Ry-King, brown	33
Ry-King, fibre plus	28
Ryvita High Fibre Crackerbread	14
Ryvita High Fibre Crispbread	23
Ryvita, brown	26
Ryvita, sesame seed	31
Slymbred rye	12

Breakfast cereals

Muesli, 'no added sugar or salt' variety	105
Porridge oats, per oz/25 g	110
Porridge, average bowl	150
Shredded Wheat, per item	75
Shreddies, per oz/25 g	95
Weetabix, per item	65
Weetaflakes, per oz/25 g	95

Cheese

All per oz/25 g

Bel Paese	95
Boursin	115
Brie	90
Camembert	90
Cottage cheese:	
Natural	27
Pineapple	24
Edam	90
Fromage frais:	
Low-fat natural	15
Natural	35
Fruit	35
Mozzarella	90
Soft cheese, skimmed milk	25
Soft cheese, medium-fat	45

Cream

All per oz/25 g

Half cream	35

Non-dairy:
    Elmlea single   55
    Shape single   32
Single   60
Soured   60

Dressings and condiments

Cornflour, per teaspoon	10
French dressing, per tablespoon	75
Garlic, garlic purée	neg
Herbs, fresh or dried	neg
Mayonnaise, per dessertspoon	80
Mayonnaise, reduced-calorie, per dessertspoon	40
Oyster sauce, per teaspoon	4
Soya sauce, per teaspoon	4
Spices, fresh or dried	neg
Vinegar	0
Worcestershire sauce, per teaspoon	4

Drinks

Beer, lager, stout, per ½ pint, average	90
Coffee, all types, no milk or sugar	0
Fruit tea, all types	neg
Herbal tea, all types	neg
Juice, per fl oz/25 ml:	
Apple	10
Grape	15
Grapefruit	10
Mixed vegetable	5

Orange	10
Peach	10
Pineapple	11
Tomato	5
Tea, no milk or sugar	0
Wine, per 5 fl oz/150 ml glass, average	90

Eggs
Raw, baked, boiled or poached (no added fat)
Per egg

Size 2	90
Size 3	80
Size 4	75

Fats, oils, low-fat spreads

Butter, per oz/25 g	210
Butter to cover 1 medium slice bread	50
Low-fat spread, per oz/25 g	105
Low-fat spread to cover 1 slice bread	15
Oil, corn, olive, sunflower, per oz/25 g	255
Per tablespoon	120
Sunflower margarine, per oz/25 g	210
Sunflower margarine to cover 1 slice bread	30

Fish
All per oz/25 g unless stated otherwise

Cod fillet, raw	20
Coley, raw	20
Crab, dressed	35

Fish cake in wholemeal crumbs, per item, grilled	80
Fish finger in wholemeal crumbs, per item, grilled	50
Haddock fillet, raw	20
Hake, raw	25
Halibut fillet, raw	30
Herring fillet, raw	65
Herring, one whole 6 oz/175 g, grilled	240
Herring roes, raw	25
Mackerel fillet, raw	60
Mackerel, one whole 8 oz/225 g, grilled	325
Monkfish, raw	20
Mullet, raw	40
Mussels, shelled	25
Oysters, each	5
Pilchards in tomato sauce	35
Plaice fillet, raw	25
Salmon, canned, drained	45
Salmon, fresh, fillet	55
Sardines, canned, drained	60
Sardines in tomato sauce	50
Scallops, raw, shelled	20
Skate fillet, raw	30
Sole fillet, raw	25
Trout fillet, raw	40
Trout, one whole 8 oz/225 g, grilled	200
Tuna, canned, drained	60

Fruit

All per item unless stated otherwise

Apple, dessert	40
Apple, cooking, per oz/25 g	10
Apricot, fresh	15
Apricot, dried, 1 oz/25 g	50
Banana, average	70
Blackberries, per oz/25 g	10
Blackcurrants, per oz/25 g	10
Cherries, per oz/25 g	10
Currants, per oz/25 g	70
Damsons, per oz/25 g	10
Date	15
Fig	30
Gooseberries, dessert, per oz/25 g	10
Gooseberries, cooking, per oz/25 g	5
Grapefruit	30
Grapes, per oz/25 g	15
Kiwifruit	30
Lemon	20
Mandarins in natural juice, per oz/25 g	10
Mango	100
Melon, 8 oz/225 g slice	30
Nectarine	40
Orange	50
Peach	50
Pear	50
Pineapple, 1 slice	25
Pineapple canned in juice, per oz/25 g	15
Plum	20

Prunes, stoned, per oz/25 g	50
Raisins, per oz/25 g	70
Raspberries, per oz/25 g	7
Rhubarb, 1 stick	5
Strawberries, per oz/25 g	7
Tangerine or satsuma	20
Sultanas, per oz/25 g	70

Ice cream
Vanilla, all varieties, average, per oz	50

Meat, poultry and game
All per oz/25 g unless stated otherwise

Beef, extra lean — roast, grilled	50
Beefburger, 1 small, grilled	100
Chicken, roast or grilled, on bone	40
Chicken, roast or grilled including skin	60
Chicken, one average joint, roast or grilled	250
Duck, wild	35
Grouse, no bone	50
Kidney, 1 whole lamb's	50
Lamb, lean fillet	50
Lamb, extra lean loin chop	200
Liver	50
Partridge, no bone	60
Pheasant, flesh only	60
Pork, lean only, roast or grilled	50
Rabbit, stewed, meat only	50
Tongue	60
Turkey, roast, meat only	40

Veal, roast or grilled   30
Veal escalope in wholemeal breadcrumbs, fried in
    corn oil, 1 average   350

Milk
Skimmed, per pint   200
Skimmed, enough for 1 average cup tea   15
Semi-skimmed, per pint   265
Whole, per pint   380

Nuts and seeds
All per oz/25g and all shelled weight
Almonds   160
Brazils   175
Cashews   160
Chestnuts   48
Coconut, fresh   100
Hazelnuts   105
Peanuts, fresh, unsalted   160
Pine kernels   180
Pumpkin seeds   175
Sesame seeds   160
Sunfower seeds   170
Walnuts   150

Pasta
Boiled, wholewheat, all kinds, per oz/25g   35
Raw, wholemeal, all kinds, per oz/25g   100

Preserves and spreads
All per oz unless otherwise stated

Honey	80
Jam, reduced-sugar	50
Marmalade, reduced-sugar	50
Pure fruit spread	30
Peanut butter	175
1 dessertspoon	70

Pulses

Baked beans, reduced sugar and salt, per oz/25 g	15
Chick peas, boiled, per oz/25 g	40
Raw, per oz/25 g	90
Kidney beans, canned or boiled, per oz/25 g	25
Raw, per oz/25 g	80
Lentils, brown or green, boiled, per oz/25 g	30
Raw, per oz/25 g	100
Lentil soup, home-made, 1 average bowl	200
Soya beans, boiled, per oz/25 g	50
Raw, per oz/25 g	110

Rice

Boiled, per oz/25 g	35
Raw per oz/25 g	100

Sugar
All kinds

Per oz/25 g	110
Per rounded teaspoonful	25

Per square lump   10

Vegetables
All per oz unless stated otherwise — raw, baked, steamed, boiled or microwaved without fat

Artichoke, globe, 1 item	10
Artichoke, Jerusalem	5
Asparagus, 1 spear	5
Aubergine	4
Avocado, half a medium	250
Beans, broad	15
Beans, French	10
Beans, runner	5
Beansprouts	5
Beetroot	12
Broccoli	5
Brussels sprouts	5
Cabbage, white, red, spring, etc	4
Carrots	5
Cauliflower	4
Celeriac	4
Celery, 1 stick	3
Chicory	3
Chinese leaves	3
Corn on the cob, 1 item	80
Courgettes	4
Cucumber	3
Fennel	5
Leek	10
Lettuce, all kinds	3

Marrow	3
Mushrooms	5
Mustard and cress, whole box	5
Onion	5
Parsnip	15
Peas, fresh or frozen	15
Pepper, sweet, any colour	4
Potato, old	25
Potato, new	22
Potato, 1 × 6 oz/175 g baked	150
Potato, instant mashed, low-salt	20
Potato chips, thick-cut, fried in corn oil	60
Potato, roast, 1 chunk	80
Radish, 1	2
Spinach	7
Swede	5
Sweetcorn	25
Sweet potato	25
Tomato	4
Tomato, 1 average whole	10
Tomato canned in juice	3
Turnip	5
Watercress	5

Vegetarian products

Nut cutlet or loaf, per oz/25 g	50
Average 5 oz/150 g	250
Soya mince, per oz/25 g	95
Tofu, drained, per oz/25 g	25
VegeBurger, one item	150

Yogurt

Yogurt, low-fat natural, per oz/25 g	15
Yogurt, fruit, per oz/25 g	25
Yogurt, Greek strained, per oz/25 g	40
Yogurt, whole milk, per oz/25 g	25
Yogurt, diet, fruit, per tub/125 g	50